I.V.F.
In Vitro Fertilisation

PROFESSOR CARL WOOD
ROBYN RILEY

I.V.F.
In Vitro Fertilisation

PROFESSOR CARL WOOD
ROBYN RILEY

HILL OF CONTENT
Melbourne

First published in Australia 1983
Revised edition 1984
Second revised edition 1987
New edition 1992

Hill of Content Publishing Co Pty Ltd
86 Bourke Street, Melbourne

© Copyright Carl Wood 1992
　　　　　　Robyn Riley 1992

Typeset in Australia by Midland Typesetters, Maryborough
Printed in Australia by Australian Print Group, Victoria
Cover design: Julian Jones
Photographs: Les O'Rourke
Back cover photograph: Fiona Hamilton

Illustrations: Gary Turner

Cataloguing-in-publication data
Wood, Carl, date
IVF (in vitro fertilisation).

3rd ed. Includes index.
ISBN 0 85572 212 6

1. Fertilisation in vitro, Human. 2. Human embryo—
Transplantation. I. Riley, Robyn, date   . II. Title.

618. 178059

ACKNOWLEDGEMENTS

Both Robyn and I would like to point out that this book has been written to give a general guide to IVF and related procedures. Each patient's symptoms and treatment is different, so this book should be used as a resource guide only.

I would like to acknowledge the help of those contributing to the development and success of the technique, to the dedicated scientists—in particular Professor Alan Trounson—technicians, and medical, nursing and administrative staff who have enabled the procedure to be carried out.

I would also like to thank Monash and Melbourne Universities, the Queen Victoria Medical Centre, the Royal Women's Hospital and Epworth Medical Centre which supported the program during the difficult stage of development, to research workers in the Howard Florey and Prince Henry's Hospital Research Institutes, and to the Ford Foundation and the National Health and Medical Research Council for financial support.

Robyn and I sincerely thank Diane Molloy and Trina King and the IMC staff who helped with information for this book. We would also like to thank Henry Sathananthan from the Lincoln Institute for allowing us to publish some of his photographs.

My thanks to my wife Marie and my family who have been understanding and patient during my involvement in the work.

Our thanks also to Anne Grendon for her considerable help in typing this book and also to Susie Andrews.

Carl Wood
Robyn Riley

CONTENTS

1	Breaking Down the Barriers (The In Vitro Fertilisation story)	1
2	What are the Causes and Treatment of Infertility? (A look at male and female infertility)	10
3	When to Proceed to IVF and GIFT	28
4	Common Questions about In Vitro Fertilisation	32
5	Telling It Like It Is (IVF patients talk about their own experiences)	39
6	The Not-So-Merry-Go-Round (The treatment cycle)	52
7	Taking Drugs	73
8	And Baby Makes Three, or Four . . . (Looking at the success rates and pregnancy)	79
9	Myths and Misconceptions	85
10	A Helping Hand (Why counselling sessions are necessary)	91
11	Facing Facts (IVF and the Law)	97
12	Answering the Critics	104
13	IVF Speak (Glossary of terms used)	110
	Index	123

CHRONOLOGY OF IVF PROCEDURES IN AUSTRALIA AND DEVELOPMENT OF INFERTILITY MEDICAL CENTRE

1971   IVF research began at Queen Victoria Medical Centre (QVMC) and Royal Women's Hospital (RWH). This was initiated by Carl Wood's appointment of Dr Alex Lopata as an embryologist. This became a joint venture between Monash and Melbourne Universities. The IVF procedure was established by Monash at QVMC. The Melbourne clinical team was at RWH.

A joint committee was chaired by Professor Carl Wood. The team members at Monash/QVMC included Carl Wood, Alex Lopata, John Leeton and Mac Talbot.

At Melbourne/RWH the team was Ian Johnston and Jim Brown.

1973   First IVF pregnancy in the world was reported by conjoint team in Melbourne and resulted in early embryo death.

1977   Ford Foundation awarded grant to Carl Wood for IVF research for three years. This enabled Alan Trounson to join the research team.

1978   First IVF birth in the world, resulting from Bob Edwards and Patrick Steptoe's pioneering work in the UK.

1979 First two sustained IVF pregnancies reported by Melbourne conjoint team in Australia.

1980 First IVF birth in Australia at RWH. Johnston, Lopata and Brown then set up own program at RWH. Monash team now Wood, Trounson, Leeton, Talbot and Kovacs.

The Infertility Medical Centre (IMC) was formed.

The IMC Clinic used a fertility drug schedule—this was one of the major steps forward in IVF technology as it increased pregnancy rates from 2% to 18% and therefore made IVF programs viable. First IMC IVF pregnancies.

1981 IMC moved to Epworth Hospital in order to expand clinical services, a joint Monash University/Epworth venture.

The Waller Committee was established to overview IVF work.

Carl Wood awarded CBE for services to IVF.

1983 Freezing of human embryos by Alan Trounson and Linda Mohr resulted in world's first frozen embryo baby at IMC.

1984 World's First Donor Egg Baby. IMC team achieved the world's first birth in a woman without ovaries, using donor eggs, the creation of an artificial menstrual cycle, and a special hormone schedule for the first 10 weeks of pregnancy.

Women who had no eggs or unsuitable eggs causing the risk of chromosomal or genetic disease were also treated.

1985 First IVF twins born from frozen embryos born in Australia.

1986 The world's first pregnancy and birth from the sperm retrieval operation performed on a patient whose vasectomy reversal had failed.

IMC helped establish IVF Australia's first IVF clinic in America.

1988   Australia's first IVF surrogate birth May, 1988. IMC announces the birth of its 500th IVF baby.

1990   IMC establishes mobile IVF clinics for Victorian country patients in Geelong, and planning clinics elsewhere in Victoria. The first pregnancies from microinjection of sperm for severe male infertility occurred.

1
BREAKING DOWN THE BARRIERS

The In-vitro fertilisation technique was developed in Australia because the infertile population was putting an enormous amount of pressure on scientists and doctors to come up with alternatives.

There were two main reasons for this. The number of children for adoption had declined markedly in the early 1970s and waiting lists for those wishing to adopt had increased dramatically.

There was also an understanding that tubal surgery was not as successful as hoped and this surgery was not restoring the tubes in many women.

We were achieving an overall success rate of about 30 per cent and surgeons were usually successful in unblocking the tube. Unfortunately, the problem is often extended beyond a simple blockage.

While surgeons can remove a blockage, they cannot restore the crucial functions of the tube. Microsurgery, first done in Australia by a Monash group, did offer some hope because it meant more gentle and accurate surgery was possible. But although the success rate improved somewhat, tubal surgery is still frequently unsuccessful.

There have been experiments with alternatives. Earlier this century, surgeons tried placing the ovary in the uterus when the tubes had been severely damaged. They hoped that fertilisation and embryo growth would occur once the egg was in the uterine cavity.

A small number of pregnancies did result using this technique but it involved considerable danger because the transferred ovary could become diseased, making its removal necessary. Also, if pregnancy did occur, the uterus was at risk of rupturing along the scar formed to facilitate the transfer of the ovary.

Another alternative was to transplant a tube from a donor. This was done by a Melbourne team I organised with Bernie O'Brien from St Vincent's Hospital in 1975. The technique was successful but the graft was rejected before a pregnancy occurred.

Although transplant procedures are technically feasible, the drugs used to suppress rejection of transplanted tissue are very toxic and most doctors will agree to their use only when life is threatened. Tubal transplants may provide a practical alternative if less toxic drugs are available to suppress rejection and the matching of donors and recipients becomes more accurate, thus minimizing the risk of rejection.

How did we develop the IVF technique?

Dr Bob Edwards, working at Cambridge University in the 1960s, started fertilising human eggs collected by Dr Patrick Steptoe. By 1970, Dr Edwards was able to achieve apparently normal embryo growth to the eight and sixteen cell stage.

In 1969 I visited Dr Neil Moore and Alan Trounson in New South Wales as I was aware that embryo culture in the laboratory was being carried out in sheep. The possibility of donor embryo transfer was suggested by Neil because this was a technique already used in the cattle industry to achieve pregnancy. The difficulty with patients was obvious as the egg would not be the patient's even if the donor was artificially inseminated with the husband's sperm. It was decided that although IVF and embryo transfer had not been achieved in sheep or other large animals, only in mice, that this would be the best alternative.

A key person was the embryologist but neither Neil Moore nor Alan Trounson were available at this time. I turned to physiologist, Alex Lopata, and asked him to start training as an embryologist.

In Melbourne, interest in the possibility of IVF among clinicians and researchers at both Queen Victoria Medical Centre (affiliated with Monash University, and where the clinical infertility work was headed by Prof John Leeton) and at the Royal Women's Hospital (affiliated with the University of Melbourne, and where the Reproductive Biology Unit was headed by Mr Ian Johnston) led to the formation of a collaborative team.

From 1970 to 1972, the Melbourne team collected eggs when operating on ovaries and also when using the technique of laparoscopy which was favoured by Dr Patrick Steptoe in England. Dr Lopata examined the eggs and devised his own criteria for assessing their ripeness and growth. This information was essential in developing the procedure.

By 1973 our work had progressed sufficiently to attempt IVF and Embryo Transfer (ET). We were delighted when two patients at the Queen Victoria Medical Centre appeared to achieve pregnancies, based on evidence from hormone tests. Although neither pregnancy progressed beyond a few days, the objective of by-passing tubal blockage seemed close. We were not to know then that it would take another seven years before a baby was born in Melbourne using the IVF and ET techniques.

Why did it take us so long to achieve that first pregnancy?

In the early 1970s, all of our patients were volunteers who had been warned that there was very little possibility they would actually get pregnant. We needed their invaluable help to develop the technique. But the main reason for our lack of early success was that the culture systems used in the laboratory were not optimum.

Dr Alan Trounson joined our team in 1976 and his work included helping us to achieve a better medium for the cultures. He did this in two ways.

One was to suggest that we would be best to check the medium with scientists working with mice embryos. Up until that time it had only been checked on human sperm.

The second was to show that some of the oil we used with the medium was toxic.

He also pointed out that one of the catheters had embryo toxins in it as well.

The work of English doctors Patrick Steptoe and Bob Edwards was also invaluable. They helped in two critical ways. Patrick Steptoe was the first to collect eggs using laparoscopy. Previously, we had been collecting eggs as far back as 1971 but this was done via an open operation.

Dr Mac Talbot worked with Patrick Steptoe to learn the technique and he brought it back to us.

Bob Edwards also helped keep our morale up because he had published the results of obtaining human embryos in the 1970s. Although this had not resulted in a pregnancy at that time, it did offer us encouragement that it was possible.

Obviously the turning point came in 1978 when Bob Edwards and Patrick Steptoe announced the birth of Louise Brown, the world's first IVF baby.

In that same year we were achieving embryo formation in 10 to 20 per cent of patients, but still could not achieve that elusive pregnancy.

Naturally we were disappointed not to be the first but we were all delighted that the birth of Louise Brown meant that the possibilities of these techniques were confirmed. IVF was possible.

By the end of 1979 success seemed imminent; many embryos were growing apparently normally in the tissue culture system. Then, a patient at the Royal Women's Hospital became pregnant.

Candice Reed—the first 'test-tube baby' success in Australia—was born in Melbourne in 1980.

Dr Alan Trounson at the Queen Victoria Medical Centre was influential in the routine use of fertility pills to stimulate egg development, the quality control system for the culture fluids, and improvements in egg ripening techniques. These measures, together with refinements in egg pick-up and embryo transfer, resulted in a series of pregnancies at the Queen Victoria Medical Centre in 1980.

Initially, the system of egg pick-ups was not very satisfactory and eggs were recovered from only 30 to 50 per cent of patients using the technique of laparoscopy. So, Dr Peter Renou, an obstetrician and gynaecologist, turned his attention to the problem. He devised a fine-gauge needle with an internal coat of teflon. This virtually eliminated the problem of eggs and embryos sticking to the fine tube and resulted in successful egg pick-ups in more than 80 per cent of patients. Members of the team also devised special catheters to facilitate the safe and gentle transfer of the embryo.

The routine use of fertility pills during the test-tube baby procedure was introduced at the Queen Victoria. Previously, Dr Edwards had abandoned the use of fertility drugs to stimulate ovulation at a predictable time, preferring to work with the natural menstrual cycle. His studies indicated that the use of fertility pills could disturb the production of hormones necessary for a successful pregnancy.

Problems of logistics, however, made it impossible to rely on the natural cycle. Ovulation can occur at any time, day or night, which necessitates access to an operating theatre with only six to 12 hours notice.

For this reason, and because we were unconvinced by Dr Edwards' finding and had access to expert advice from Dr Jim Brown on hormone responses to induced ovulation, we persevered with the fertility pill. This approach seemed reasonable since pregnancy often follows the use of fertility pills in women who are not ovulating and therefore the use of such pills should be compatible with IVF. This was shown to be true and all early successes at the Queen Victoria Medical Centre followed use of fertility pills.

Another advantage of this approach was that two or more eggs usually ripened in the ovaries instead of only one. This improved the chance of picking up several ripe eggs, and increased the chance of producing one or more embryos for transfer.

Subsequently we have found that the likelihood of pregnancy is greater for the transfer of three embryos (30 per cent) than for two embryos (23 per cent) which again is greater than for one (12 per cent). Transferring four embryos does not increase the success rate further.

Several other discoveries proved to be important.

For some years it was thought that ripening of an immature egg in the laboratory was an impossibility. We discovered that by leaving the eggs for five or six hours in the culture fluid prior to the addition of sperm cells, embryo development was enhanced. Using a high-powered electron microscope, Dr Henry Sathananthan of the Lincoln Institute in Melbourne was able to demonstrate physical differences, indicating greater maturity, in eggs left alone in the culture fluid for six hours, in comparison with those examined after pick-up.

Previous attempts at fertilisation of immature eggs demonstrated a high rate of failed or incomplete fertilisation. Now, maturing eggs for four to six hours before the addition of sperm cells has become routine practice, and has resulted in a significantly increased success rate in embryo formation.

Similar work by Dr Edwards has confirmed this finding and occasionally he has left eggs up to 18 hours before adding sperm cells.

Originally, the culture fluid used for growing the eggs and embryos was extremely complex, containing more than 180 different substances. This 'broth' contained most of the constituents of the serum portion of human blood and had been used for many years to culture animal eggs and embryos. The disadvantage of working with such a highly complex fluid is that it is unclear which of the ingredients are essential for success and which are unnecessary extras. And in the situation where the fluid fails to promote growth, it is difficult to pinpoint the chemical error or errors responsible.

We found with considerable relief that fertilisation and normal embryo growth were possible when using much more simple culture fluids which contained only 10 to 20 different substances and could be prepared in our own laboratory. By removing inessential substances from the culture fluids, we gained valuable insights into the vital ingredients for egg and embryo growth and into the building blocks of early life. One thing is certain - it is easy for toxic chemicals to gain access to the culture fluid and inhibit growth; despite thorough washing and cleaning of laboratory apparatus, substances can pass into the fluid from glass and plastic tubes.

One change that became necessary during 1980 and 1981 had more to do with logistics than techniques. The clinical work of the program was transferred to St Andrew's Hospital at the edge of Melbourne's central business district. This was because of demands for theatre time and the necessity of ready access to hospital beds.

In 1982 this arrangement was replaced by a new Monash University Infertility Service at Epworth Hospital, also on the fringe of central Melbourne, which was established in order to increase the efficiency of treating the 2000 couples on the waiting list.

Meanwhile, the basic research continued at the Queen Victoria Medical Centre, and scientists from more than twenty countries visited Melbourne to learn the techniques involved.

Where did we go from here?
Freezing Embryos

One of the most important advances in IVF in recent years is the development of cryopreservation (freezing) techniques. This allowed preservation and later use of excess embryos which could not be transferred in the treatment cycle. Alan Trounson and his team developed the freezing technique, which was adapted from the successful techniques used for cattle and sheep embryos.

The first frozen embryo baby in the world was born at Queen Victoria Medical Centre in 1984.

That technique is now more efficient today. It has been further modified with the introduction of different chemical preservants.

Alan is also carrying out experiments on using an ultra-rapid freezing technique.

When we started using the freezing technique, the survival rate was only five per cent. It is now, per embryo, eight per cent, but most couples elect to have two or three embryos put back so most transfers have a success rate of around 15-18 per cent.

One in three embryos do not survive cryopreservation, the cells of the embryos disintegrate. Successful freezing depends partly on the quality of the embryo. The actual physics and chemistry of cryopreservation is not yet fully understood.

Egg Freezing

Freezing eggs offers many possibilities. When a woman is undergoing premature menopause or develops ovarian cancer, we hope to be able to retrieve eggs and freeze them until these women are able and wish to use them.

We have been trying to freeze eggs for some time. It is difficult because of the risk of chromosomal abnormalities. In the mature egg, chromosomes are on a spindle inside the cell. When they are in this stage they are unstable so that when the egg is frozen, the chromosomes "slip off" the spindle and this creates obvious problems. Although two babies have resulted from this technique, the risks of the present methods have prevented further use.

Perhaps the solution will lie in us succeeding to retrieve immature 'unripe' eggs. The unripe egg has the chromosomes in a much more stable state, and is less liable to chromosome damage.

Unripe eggs have not reached day 12 of the cycle. In 1990, a Korean group reported that they could ripen unripe eggs in the laboratory, and then fertilise them to produce embryos. We have repeated this work successfully.

We also need to freeze and store these unripe eggs. Sounds simple? It is not. But Alan Trounson believes that technically it will be possible to freeze unripe eggs. I believe that we will be able to retrieve and freeze unripe eggs. But obviously we have a lot of work to do.

Another advantage of egg freezing would be to those women who have decided to delay their childbearing because of their career and who do not want to risk having a child with Down's Syndrome by becoming pregnant when they are over the age of 37 years. Egg storage may also be an insurance against developing infertility in future years.

What may be possible is for women to have unripe eggs retrieved when they are in their early 20s, and "stored" until they are ready to use them.

Another benefit of maturing eggs would be for those women having laparoscopies as part of infertility investigations to have the unripe eggs collected at this time. The eggs could be frozen or matured and inseminated with the husband's sperm. This may avoid a stimulation cycle or an IVF or GIFT program.

So there is a big incentive to succeed with this technique.

Donor Eggs

Donor eggs have also been an important development. We achieved the world's first "donor-egg" baby in 1984 and this offered much promise and hope for those women who, through disease or congenital abnormalities, do not have ovaries. It also helped those women who had undergone premature menopause.

First, we worked out how to produce an artificial menstrual cycle. We did this by using a combination of the two main hormones that the ovary produces—oestrogen and progesterone.

We then checked that their blood levels matched those of women in a natural cycle who had their own ovaries.

We also took specimens from the lining of their uterus to make sure the uterus was responding to these hormones.

We used unknown donors on the IVF program who had too many eggs and who were happy to donate them to other women. The eggs were "donated" to a patient who had been on oestrogen for anywhere between 12 and 18 days to prepare the lining of the uterus. The donated eggs were placed with the husband's sperm and the embryo transferred to the tube or uterus of the infertile woman.

After this, progesterone was given to maintain a possible pregnancy. We then had the problem of not knowing exactly how long to continue the hormone treatments. A pregnancy is normally supported by the ovaries until the sixth to eighth week. After that, the placenta takes over the hormonal support.

It turned out that the recipient of the donor egg would need progesterone for at least six weeks until the placenta could take over. We achieved a pregnancy the first time we used the technique.

From this we learnt that you only need two hormones—oestrogen and progesterone—to support a pregnancy.

This also helped us in understanding natural abortions because we now know that if the oestrogen and progesterone levels drop early in the pregnancy there is no support mechanism and a pregnancy is no longer viable.

Since then, the donor egg program has had an interesting history. The Government placed a moratorium on the use of donor eggs but not on donor sperm.

The patients on our program at the time heard about the moratorium and went to the Equal Opportunity Board to lodge a complaint. A few days before the hearing, the moratorium was lifted and the case withdrawn.

One patient conceived before the moratorium was put in place and when we announced the pregnancy it caused a few ripples because members of the media accused us of going against the moratorium.

This was not the case. Our pregnancy was established before the moratorium was put in place.

We are also now allowed to use known or unknown donor eggs and sperm which has been a major step forward. Infertile couples are the legal parents of the child and the donor has no claim on the child. Nor has the child a claim on the donor. Details of social, education and physical characteristics of the donor are given to the parents to inform the child about their biological parent.

Obviously, if you are using known donors, the process is much quicker because there is no waiting. The known donor gives all her eggs to the couple and the success rate per treatment is highest of all procedures 30-40 per cent.

In the following chapters I have endeavoured to explain in more detail the many options now available to infertile couples.

I have also discussed the many myths and misunderstandings surrounding IVF and hope to allay any fears or concerns patients may have.

2
WHAT ARE THE CAUSES AND TREATMENT OF INFERTILITY?

By the time you enter an IVF program, you will be aware of these words: infertility, sub-fertility or sterility.

Infertility means an inability to conceive: sub-fertility is sometimes used to describe a reduced state of fertility and sterility means that one can never conceive.

Most people entering the program have already had one year or more of regular unprotected intercourse before infertility was diagnosed.

Why do we choose one year as a guide? About 85 to 90 per cent of "normal, healthy" couples become pregnant within this time, 50 per cent after about five months of regular intercourse.

Most couples who have failed to conceive within this time will start investigations by visiting their general practitioner. He or she will probably organise a semen check for the male and temperature charts or blood tests for the female to establish if ovulation is occurring.

The next step is a referral to a specialist for further investigations.

The woman may have a laparoscopy to determine the presence of endometriosis, pelvic inflammatory disease or tubal disease or a hysteroscopy to make sure the uterus is normal. Vaginal swabs to check for infection and a check on sperm movement in the cervix may also be necessary. It is sensible for the husband to have undergone a semen analysis before the partner undergoes these tests. Antibody tests in the semen may detect another cause of infertility.

There are a number of factors that may have contributed to an increased risk of infertility.

FEMALE INFERTILITY

One of the most common causes of infertility is tubal disease.

The use of the intrauterine device (IUD) is associated occasionally with infection and irreversible damage to the fallopian tubes, and the use of the Pill—in place of the condom which acts as a barrier to the sexually transmitted organisms that may cause infertility—may have resulted in an increased risk of sexually transmitted diseases.

The greater availability of abortion may have resulted in an increased incidence of infertility either because of infection of the fallopian tubes or because of damage to the cervix resulting in an inability to maintain a pregnancy.

The trend to postpone the first pregnancy may also contribute to infertility because when a woman delays starting a family, she may have an increased risk of developing pelvic infection or endometriosis.

The more frequent use of condoms, the increased awareness of women concerning the risks of pelvic infection and the more ready use of diagnostic tests and antibiotics by medical practitioners has controlled these risks.

Pelvic Inflammatory Disease (PID)

One of the first questions many couples ask is could they have prevented their infertility? About 25 per cent of infertility can be prevented. Pelvic Inflammatory Disease (PID) is one disease that may be prevented.

It is a major health problem affecting women and is sexually transmitted in a large number of cases.

Gynaecological and obstetrical procedures are another cause.

We find that PID is usually accompanied by symptoms which may include lower abdominal pain, painful or irregular periods, deep discomfort at intercourse, vaginal discharge, fever and frequent and painful emptying of the bladder. These symptoms could also be a pointer to endometriosis.

Women at risk for PID are usually those under 25 years, those with several sexual partners, those not using the barrier methods of contraception and those undergoing gynaecological procedures such as insertion of an IUD or a curettage.

Any of the above symptoms should be discussed with your doctor.

As the risk of pelvic infection is sometimes higher among users of IUDs, this form of contraception may not be suitable for women who have not completed their families. If you have had an IUD inserted and you are experiencing pain or an unpleasant discharge, this may indicate infection and you should talk to your doctor immediately.

Possible alternatives are condoms and vaginal diaphragms which produce adequate but less effective protection. These are used with spermicidal preparations which also reduce the risk of infection.

For women with new sexual partners, routine check-ups are advisable, particularly for chlamydia and gonorrhoea. These involve a physical examination of the pelvis and taking swabs to check for potentially harmful bacteria.

Endometriosis

Another common cause of infertility is endometriosis. This is a condition where the lining of the uterus (endometrium) is found growing in areas other than the uterus.

Because the tissue is the same as that found in the uterus, it responds to the same hormones which affect the menstrual cycle. During the menstrual period these deposits of tissue also bleed. But this blood goes straight into the abdomen and cannot escape like menstrual fluid. The cause of endometriosis is still not known nor is there a permanent cure yet. Naturally there are many theories.

Some believe that it is caused by fragments of endometrium passing up the fallopian tubes and out into the cavity. Another theory is that it is the remnants of the woman's foetal tissue inside the abdomen responding to the ovarian hormones.

Why some women develop endometriosis and others do not is not fully understood. We know that it can occur in any woman who menstruates and can occur at any time from the onset of puberty through to menopause.

The most likely explanation is that endometrial cells from menstrual fluid spill back through the tubes into the abdomen and grow in the pelvis. The immune defence is unable to cope with these cells which implant and grow as a result. The cells, mobilised to deal with the endometrial cells, may produce chemicals which reduce sperm motility and embryo growth. When the disease is severe, mechanical blockage of tubes or displacement of ovaries add to problems causing infertility.

Symptoms can include cyclical pain at ovulation, premenstrual or menstrual phase, changes in bowel or bladder function, bloating, tiredness, sexual pain and premenstrual tension. The disease can also cause excessive or irregular menstrual flow, brown discharge, infertility, adhesions and ovarian cysts (chocolate cysts). Diagnosis is best made by laparoscopy. Some women experience many symptoms. Others have few or none at all.

This is why a laparoscopy is the only definite method of telling if a patient has this disease.

(A laparoscopy is a procedure under general anaesthetic in which an instrument called a laparoscope is passed into the abdomen. Patients are usually only required to stay in hospital as a day patient after this procedure.) Chemical tests done on blood may soon help in diagnosis and treatment.

Many women do not discover they have endometriosis until they start investigations for infertility.

Failure to Ovulate

Another common cause of infertility is anovulation—the failure to ovulate. This results from imbalance or inadequate production of those hormones causing ovulation, the pituitary hormones, Follicle Stimulating Hormone, Luteinizing Hormone and Prolactin, or inability of the ovary to respond to these hormones. Anovulation may be associated with being over or underweight, having excess hair growth or breast secretion, excessive exercise or stress.

Measurement of ovary and pituitary hormones and vaginal ultrasound will determine the cause and best treatment for failed ovulation.

TREATMENT

Tubal Disease

Antibiotics are used as active infection may cause temporary blockage.

Permanent blockage may be overcome by hydrotubation (the flushing of fluid through the tubes to check they are open) at the time of laparoscopy.

Blockage at the inner end of the tube may be opened by passing a catheter or balloon from the uterus with the aid of an intrauterine telescope called the hysteroscope.

Blockage at the outer end of the tube can be dealt with by surgery at the time of laparoscopy, although pregnancy rates are low, 20–30per cent.

Open surgery is advised frequently when the tubes are blocked. The overall pregnancy rate following surgery to the tubes is only about 30 per cent, or 40 per cent if microsurgery is used, but in certain types of tubal repair, such as reversal of clip sterilisation, the success rate may be much higher, 70 to 90 per cent, while when tubal disease is severe the success rate is considerably lower— 10 to 20 per cent.

In reversal operations, the portion of the tube damaged by sterilisation is cut out and the ends are re-joined. In general, the success rate of reversal depends on the length of healthy tube remaining. If only a few millimetres of tube have been damaged by the placement of a clip, then the success rate may be as high as 80 per cent, but if more than half of the tube has been damaged by the sterilisation procedure, the success rate of reversal varies from 10 to 40 per cent.

Sometimes the blockage in the tube is at the outer end where the fimbriae—the finger-like fronds nearest the ovary—are stuck together by adhesions. Using microsurgery, adhesions can be dissected away, thus allowing a passage through which the eggs can enter the tube.

Fibroids

Fibroids may require treatment if they grow into the cavity of the uterus or cause excessive bleeding or pain.

Myomectomy may be done by hysteroscopy, laparoscopy or open operation, depending on the size and site of the fibroid in the uterus. The fibroids may be reduced in size before surgery, using a hormone similar to gonadotrophin releasing hormone.

Endometriosis

If endometriosis is responsible for infertility then drug therapy, either alone or in combination with surgery, is available.

When the disease is mild, use of the drug Danazol (Danocrine, trade name) or progestogens (progesterone-like drugs) may be sufficient. But if the endometriosis has caused large cysts or nodules, particularly if this has affected the ovaries, surgery—as well as drug treatment—is usually required. GnRH agonists, such as lupron are effective, and have fewer side effects than Danazol.

Sometimes it is clear that drug therapy will not cure the endometriosis. Drugs act by reducing the production and blocking the action of the female hormone oestrogen, so reducing growth of endometrial tissue, which is the basic component of the disease process. Surgery may involve laparoscopy diathermy or laser treatment, or open surgery removing grossly diseased organs, such as the tube or ovary.

If the disease is not severe the best treatment is laparoscopy surgery done at the time of diagnosis. Pregnancy rates are as good as drug therapy and this approach avoids the delay in trying to conceive and the side effects of drugs. Some patients do not respond to drug therapy.

Treatment of endometriosis is a complicated affair and considerable explanation, supervision and counselling is required so that the best result is obtained in the shortest time, and also so that any recurrence of endometriosis is recognised at an early stage. Some patients with moderate to severe endometriosis do not respond well to IVF treatment - so the disease is usually treated before IVF therapy starts. The GIFT procedure may be effective even when the disease is active.

Hormonal causes

The treatment of hormonal causes of infertility requires identification of the hormone abnormality, the most common treatment for which involves the use of fertility pills.

If ovulation is not occurring, Clomiphene is often used. This drug stimulates the release of Follicle Stimulating Hormone (FSH) and Luteinizing Hormone (LH), and is given usually from the third or fifth to seventh or ninth day or the menstrual cycle. The dosage, which varies from one to four tablets daily, is calculated on the basis of whether ovulation returns, as determined by temperature or mucous charting, or blood measurements of the hormone progesterone.

If Clomiphene does not produce the desired response, pituitary hormones such as Human Chorionic Gonadotrophin or human pituitary extracts of the same hormones may be given. These substitute for FSH and LH.

If the infertility problem is caused by excess production of the hormone prolactin, the drug Bromocriptine (trade name, Parlodel) may be given. This is used every day and the dose is increased gradually until the level of prolactin is reduced to normal.

Ovulation, menstruation and pregnancy often follow the use of fertility drugs, but they may have some side-effects. If the ovaries are over-stimulated, pain may occur or cysts may form in the ovaries. If pain occurs when these drugs are being taken, they should be discontinued and a doctor consulted. Cysts usually disappear without other treatment.

Another problem arises if the dose of the fertility drug is too great, resulting in multiple pregnancies. For this reason the response to the drugs must be monitored carefully.

New hormone preparations are improving the treatment of hormone disorders. Gonadotrophin-releasing hormone may be used to stimulate pituitary hormone release or GnRH agonists prescribed to correct a pituitary hormone imbalance. (It exerts its effect by blocking hormone production.) Other hormones can then be used to produce artificial but balanced pituitary function.

GnRH is given to women with underactive pituitary glands and is usually administered by a subcutaneous injection using a small pump carried on the body.

Cervical Mucous

Antibiotics may cure the problem if incompatibility between the sperm and the cervical mucous is due to infection, but treatment is more difficult if antibody formation immobilises sperm cells. Intrauterine insemination with a partner's sperm cells has been tried but may not be successful because the antibodies may be present also in uterine fluid.

Treatments previously recommended to overcome the problem of antibody formation involved several months of either sexual abstinence, or the use of a condom to eliminate contact between the semen and the vagina. The rationale was that antibody production would decline with the elimination of contact; but the results of these treatment methods have proved disappointing. Suppression of antibody response with drugs such as Cortisone has some risks but has met with limited success.

At present, couples with antibody problems are being treated by In Vitro Fertilisation because if the sperm cells can penetrate the egg in the laboratory, it may by possible to by-pass the antibodies present in the female genital tract. Pregnancies have resulted.

The procedures of In Vitro Fertilisation and Embryo Transfer and Gamete Intra Fallopian Transfer are making possible the promising form of treatment which is described in detail in the following chapters.

MALE INFERTILITY

But let us not forget that males also experience fertility problems.

Temporary/reversible infertility

There are reasons you may have a poor semen sample even though you may be fertile. These include: acute illness such as influenza, infection, smoking (may affect movement of sperm), excess alcohol, some drugs (anti-cancer, anti-hypertensives, sulphasalazine), poor ejaculation (anxiety, stress, marijuana, alcohol, extreme heat/cold).

If these factors are present, then a repeat semen sample is checked three months after removing the suspected problem. It may take this time for sperm production to recover.

If none of these factors are present or the sample is still low after health is normal, you will need further checks and careful assessment.

Major causes

It the testicles are small, production may be poor. Because there is damage to the cells producing sperm, little can be done to improve the semen. The doctor will check the size of the testicles and blood tests may confirm damage to the testis. (FSH, a pituitary hormone, is high). Even normal testicle size can be associated with marked damage. Blockage in the delivery of sperm from the testis may result from infection or absence of the tubes normally delivering semen.

The presence of cancer, either in the testes or elsewhere, may impair sperm production. Anti-cancer drugs used during treatment may damage the sperm-producing cells of the testes. Therefore it is now accepted medical practice to collect and freeze some sperm prior to treatment with anti-cancer drugs. If a child is desired later, this may be achieved by artificial insemination after thawing the husband's sperm cells.

Another type of infertility in men results from the sterilisation procedure, vasectomy. Although vasectomy reversal is often successful in surgical terms, the quality of sperm cells after reversal may be unsatisfactory. Because of this, men who have been sterilised should be advised that the reversal may not succeed and before deciding to have a vasectomy, serious consideration should be given to having some sperm cells frozen. About one per cent of men who are sterilised request a reversal, usually after the death of a child or following remarriage.

If there is a failure of hormone production (FSH, LH), which is rare, this can be substituted to help produce sperm.

Nothing can be done to help infertility where there are chromosomal disorders. This test is done on men with poor semen. They may require the male hormone testosterone to improve health and sexual desire.

Undescended testes need to be treated by the time a child is five to avoid damage to the testes. Hormones and sometimes surgery are used before this age to cure the condition.

Varicose veins around the testis may affect the production of normal sperm.

Antibodies may be attached to sperm and could affect their ability to swim through the neck of the uterus (cervix) or fertilise the egg. Four months treatment with prednisolone gives a 20 per cent chance of pregnancy. However, prednisolone may produce serious complications.

Apart from the health or otherwise of the sperm cells, the ability to ejaculate is an important factor in achieving a pregnancy. This ability is difficult to assess. Any laboratory analysis of the semen requires the man to ejaculate a sample into a jar. However, the stress of masturbating in the laboratory may adversely affect the ejaculation performance.

A post coital test will determine whether sperm have been deposited in the vagina. Special condoms are available, which don't harm the sperm, for men who can't masturbate.

Intercourse occurs under a variety of conditions and ejaculation may be less effective in association with anxiety, fatigue, marijuana or excess alcohol.

Treatment

Treatment for male infertility depends upon the cause.

Temporary suppression of sperm production is overcome by removing the causal factor and waiting two to three months. Drugs for cancer may produce permanent damage while drugs used in ulcerative colitis, hypertension or leprosy usually have only temporary effects. Avoidance of temperature extremes may help sperm production, e.g. saunas, cold weather swimming.

Viral infections which inhibit sperm production are short lived and recovery can be expected in three months. While stress, smoking and alcohol may affect fertility in some men their effect can only be assessed by trial withdrawal of the insult.

Operations for varicose veins in the scrotum may improve sperm quality but the result is uncertain.

Hormones may assist men who lack pituitary hormone, a rare occurrence.

Cortisone may help men with sperm antibodies but the dose required creates risks of bone damage and the drug has to be used carefully.

Blockage in the genital tract may be overcome by microsurgery bypassing the block, usually at the level of the epididymis. Even if the blockage cannot be overcome sperm can be collected close to the blocked site and used for IVF.

Artificial insemination of the husband's sperm may be useful if the husband has a sexual problem, e.g. impotence, paraplegia, or ejaculates into the bladder, and is sometimes successful for men with low sperm characteristics.

IVF or GIFT are the best options for most men with permanent low quantity or quality sperm. The pregnancy rate per treatment ranges from 7–25 per cent, depending upon the severity of the problem.

IVF may not succeed for severe male problems—sperm counts less than 1 million per ml, less than 10 per cent motile sperm or only 10 per cent normal shaped sperm.

Microinjection of 1–3 sperm under the shell of the egg, or weakening of the shell by physical or chemical means may assist men with severe problems. A number of pregnancies have resulted from this technique.

Donor insemination is an option for couples where there is no sperm or where IVF and other treatments have failed.

Couples can choose known or unknown donors and donors are checked for genetic and sexually transmitted diseases. Information about the donor can be given to the infertile couple, excluding the donor's identity. In Victoria the law states that the infertile couples are the legal parents and the donor has no claim on the child. Counselling is given to couples before entering treatment. The success rate is about 75 per cent after nine treatments. Most pregnancies occur in the first four treatments. Donor sperm using the GIFT procedure should be considered after four to five failed treatments.

There is no increase in the risk of abnormalities in children resulting from donor insemination.

UNEXPLAINED INFERTILITY

This means infertility for which no cause has been found after extensive tests. It is also referred to as "idiopathic".

We find some 10 to 20 per cent of all infertile couples experience unexplained infertility.

This is frustrating for the couples involved because no abnormal factors are present, yet they are still unable to conceive.

The woman has normal looking tubes and ovaries and ovulation has been confirmed.

The male has had a normal semen analysis and yet pregnancy can still not be guaranteed.

Naturally, it is somewhat easier to accept if you know there is a reason for your infertility because you then know you have a specific problem and can deal with it. Unfortunately, for those with unexplained infertility, there are no answers. The most likely explanations are minor tubal disease, inability of the egg to pass from the ovary to the tube and adverse chemical factors preventing sperm transport and fertilisation.

Perhaps this is because unexplained infertility is not well known in the community and there is always the stigma attached by lay people that "you need a holiday" or "you are not doing it right". Let me say here that sexual difficulties are a very rare cause of unexplained infertility.

In couples with no obvious cause of infertility (idiopathic infertility), treatments are sometimes offered in the hope that they may overcome some unidentified factor causing the problem.

Clomiphene is often used for six months in an attempt to ensure that ovulation is occurring regularly, and that adequate hormone levels following ovulation are maintained to make certain that any embryo formed encounters a suitable uterine environment in which to grow and develop. Clomiphene has an anti-fertility effect, however, altering the cervical mucous such that it impedes sperm penetration. Super-ovulation, using drugs such as gonadotrophins, may be a preferable treatment strategy. Pregnancy rates of 10–12 per cent per cycle can be expected.

Intrauterine insemination of sperm may also result in pregnancy, with a low success rate, about 5–6 percent per treatment.

Bromocriptine has been used also when the cause of infertility is in doubt, but it is uncertain whether it is helpful to reduce normal levels of the prolactin hormone to very low levels. In view of uncertainties about the precise role of prolactin in conception, this treatment is thought to be ineffective.

It is important for couples with unknown causes of infertility to be aware that 40 per cent will become pregnant in the third or fourth year of so-called infertility. And even after this time, pregnancy may still occur.

The Gift procedure is best for couples with idiopathic infertility, the success rate per treatment being 30 per cent. One reason it is effective is that the sperm and egg are placed where fertilisation occurs so that failures of sperm or egg transport are overcome.

INFERTILITY TESTS

The tests which are carried out on a couple faced with a fertility problem depend on the couple's physical examination and medical history. The fertility specialist is the best person to decide which tests should be performed and in what sequence they should be done.

These tests include:

Hormone Assay

The ability to measure levels of progesterone, oestrogen, prolactin, testosterone, FSH (Follicle Stimulating Hormone) and LH (Luteinizing Hormone) is a valuable tool for investigation of infertility problems in both males and females.

The levels of FSH, LH and prolactin are measured by sophisticated laboratory equipment and this test can be performed on one blood sample. The results are available within one week. The test is to determine that all the levels are within normal limits and are in balance.

The blood sample is usually collected one week after expected ovulation, i.e. ovulation day 14, collection day 21. If ovulation is not occurring it can be corrected with the use of ovarian stimulating drugs.

LH Surge

A rise in LH hormone occurs 36 hours before ovulation. This can be detected by a urine test using a kit obtained from the chemist.

For couples having infrequent coitus this may be helpful.

Basal Body Temperature Chart

The charting of the basal body temperature is the traditional method of indicating if and when ovulation is occurring.

On waking, a woman takes her temperature orally or vaginally for three or four minutes before getting out of bed, talking, drinking or eating. She carefully records this in her temperature chart.

If ovulation occurs, a woman's temperature will normally rise by one degree Fahrenheit or 0.4 to 0.6 degree Centigrade during the second half of the menstrual cycle. However, the temperature is recorded on all days of the cycle and the resulting pattern observed.

The chart can indicate whether or not ovulation is occurring and changes in the temperature pattern provide an indication of the effectiveness of treatment. A prolonged rise in the basal temperature maybe the first clear indication that pregnancy has been achieved.

Mucous

Mucous changes in the cervix may be detected in the vagina. The fertile phase can be detected by the presence of an increased amount of mucous which is stretchable.

Hysterosalpingogram

This X-ray is used to check both tubal patency and the internal structure of the uterus. It is a relatively simple test which may involve discomfort for the patient. It has to be carried out in an X-ray Department. However, in order to show up the soft tissue a radio opaque dye is injected through the cervix. Some patients may feel a sensation of discomfort and cramping when this procedure is carried out.

This test is done less frequently as laparoscopy provides more accurate and more detailed information.

A series of X-ray pictures is then taken for later examination. Normally the dye will fill the uterine cavity and spill into both the fallopian tubes, then out at the ends where it will collect in the peritoneal cavity. If the dye fails to pass into the tube it may indicate a blockage or temporary spasm. The test enables the doctor to pinpoint the site of a tubal obstruction (if any) and also allows him to see any uterine defects which may be present. Some doctors believe the test can have a therapeutic effect but this is very difficult to quantify.

Laparoscopy

A laparoscopy is one of the most important tests carried out in fertility investigation. The purpose of this test is to allow the specialist to visualise the ovaries, fallopian tubes and the uterus. In order to carry out a laparoscopy, the woman has to be hospitalised usually for 2-12 hours, the procedure usually being done under a general anaesthetic. A laparoscope is a thin telescope-like instrument which is passed through a small incision in the abdomen wall near the navel.

The abdomen has first to be distended by blowing in carbon dioxide to ensure a certain amount of space exists between the organs; the laparoscope is then passed through the incision. It is possible to examine the size, shape and contours of the organs contained in the pelvic cavity. In this way adhesions, scarring, endometriosis or fibroids can be detected.

Examinations of the fimbriated ends of the fallopian tubes for adhesions can be checked to ensure they are capable of free movement. The patency of the tubes is tested by the injection of a dye into the cervix to see if any passes out through the tubes. The laparoscope may avoid the need for major abdominal surgery. Ovarian cysts, adhesions, endometriosis and fibromyomata may all be treated by operating at laparoscopy—several extra small cuts, 3-5mm, are made to pass scissors, laser or diathermy probes. The after-effects of the procedure are minimal and the scar which remains is so small as to be almost undetectable.

Dilatation and curettage is usually performed at the same time as a laparoscopy, for diagnostic purposes.

After a laparoscopy, it is normal for women to experience aching shoulders, sore chest and bloated abdomen. This results from the use of carbon dioxide gas injected into the abdomen at the beginning of the operation. This gas causes an irritation of the diaphragm which causes shoulder and chest soreness and sometimes vomiting.

Hysteroscopy

This examines the inside of the uterus. Polyps, fibroids, adhesions and bands can be detected which can also be treated at the time of hysteroscopy.

Vaginal Ultrasound

This may show fibroids, polyps, cysts, an abnormal uterus or follicle (egg) development.

Endometrial Biopsy or Dilatation & Curettage (D&C)

This test involves the microscopic examination of a scraping from the endometrium - the lining of the womb. This enables an assessment to be made of the influence of the hormone, progesterone, on the endometrium.

Progesterone causes regular and predictable changes in the structure of the lining of the womb, so microscopic evaluation is useful. Adequate levels of progesterone are essential for the critical phase of embryo implantation.

Post Coital Test

This is the observation of sperm within the cervical mucous following intercourse. The test is usually performed mid-cycle when the mucous is clear and copious, or you may be given oestrogen tablets to help produce mucous, so that when the test is performed you will be sure of having enough mucous. The couple are asked to have intercourse at home 4 to 12 hours prior to the test.

The test is a simple one, similar to a smear test except some mucous is collected from the cervix and then examined microscopically to see if live sperm are penetrating the mucous and to assess the amount of movement. If the sperm are all moving well, it is reasonable to say this test was normal.

Kremer Test (or Sperm Invasion Tests)

This test is exactly the same as the post coital test except the couple do not have intercourse. Instead a specimen of both mucous and sperm are collected and in the laboratory they are tested together for penetration at regular intervals over six hours, enabling accurate all-round assessment. The samples are also checked against donor sperm and donor mucous to help pinpoint whether a problem is in the sperm or the mucous.

Cervical pH (Acidity)

Recently there have been studies on cervical pH which can change in the cervical canal. The low pH levels indicate an acid mucous, which destroys the sperm and prevents penetration of the mucous. This is a simple test which is usually performed at the time of post coital or Kremer test. Research has gone on to alter the cervical pH levels and your doctor would be able to instruct you on the treatment necessary.

Semen Analysis

The semen analysis is the easiest, cheapest and most convenient of all fertility tests. It enables a doctor to see whether there are sperm present, how many sperm are present (the count), how many are moving (the motility) and how well they are moving and how many normal sperm there are (the morphology). Other parts of the assessment are the volume, the number of sperm alive, whether there is an infection in the reproductive tract and if there are any sperm antibodies present. All of these results give the doctor a guide to a man's potential for fertility. There is no one factor that is indicative of fertility in the semen analysis. As the sperm are produced over a 10 week period, many factors can influence their production. At the Infertility Medical Centre, semen samples can be either produced at home, or can be produced at the Centre in the Andrology laboratory in specially provided private rooms. Those produced at the Centre have the advantage of the sample being fresh when tested. However, if you feel uncomfortable about this, sample jars are available so you can produce the sample at home.

Several questions are always asked when you produce your samples. The questions and reasons why are as follows:

1 **Time of collection?** Changes in the sperm quality may occur with time. A delay of more than one hour may harm the specimen.
2 **Transport temperature?** Low or high temperatures may affect the sperm motility.
3 **Number of days of abstinence?** This may affect the semen volume and the sperm numbers, especially if it is less than three days.
4 **Method of collection?** The sample is usually collected by masturbation. Special condoms are available for men who cannot masturbate. These samples are satisfactory.
5 **Was the complete sample collected?** If any of the sample was missed, this will give misleading results, particularly as the first part of the ejaculate contains most of the sperm.
6 **Have you been ill recently?** A cold or flu can affect the sperm quality. Serious illnesses within the past few months may also affect the sample.
7 **Are you taking any medication?** Some medications can cause variability in the semen analysis. Other drugs can make it difficult to produce the specimen.

It is always assumed that what you produce is representative of your usual semen analysis. If you feel that there has been anything wrong in the collection of the sample, you should always let one of the lab staff know.

3
WHEN TO PROCEED TO IVF AND GIFT

When a couple is sterile, e.g. a woman has no tubes, IVF may be proceeded to as soon as pregnancy is desired.

When pregnancy is possible but delayed beyond the normal time taken to conceive, IVF or GIFT can be considered. The average time to conceive is five months and ten to fifteen per cent of couples are not pregnant after one year. Most couples seek treatment after nine to fifteen months of infertility. If you are over 40 years, treatment is more urgent as only 25 per cent of couples will achieve pregnancy in one year. Age and the strength of desire to conceive will determine when you seek treatment.

IVF or GIFT are indicated when other simpler treatments have failed or when there is no other treatment e.g. men with low sperm qualities and testicular damage.

GIFT is the preferred treatment for women with normal tubes because the success rate is at least 30 per cent per treatment, 50-100 per cent higher than IVF. Endometriosis, unknown factor infertility, minor tubal damage, and mild to moderate male infertility are all candidates for GIFT. It works because the sperm and egg(s) are placed in the normal place where fertilisation occurs, so neither the sperm nor the eggs have to travel to this site. Also the tubal environment is the natural site for fertilisation and embryo development, and so far is superior to the laboratory where IVF occurs.

IVF is indicated in tubal disease or in severe male infertility when it is important to know whether the sperm can fertilise the egg. This is not possible in the GIFT procedure unless pregnancy occurs or excess eggs are available to combine IVF and GIFT.

The tubal problems include women with blocked tubes, no tubes, repeated ectopic pregnancies and failed tubal surgery. While most tubal damage results from infection, some occurs as a result of endometriosis or previous surgery.

Other treatments are used less often and involve starting off with IVF and then transferring the fertilised egg (pronuclear embryo) or dividing embryo to the tube. These procedures are called PROST (pronuclear stage transfer) or ZIFT (zygote intra fallopian tube) for single cell embryo transfer, or TEST (tubal embryo stage transfer) which usually means transfer of the embryo after division to the 2, 4 or 8 cell stage. These procedures are used by clinics that prefer IVF initially to determine whether fertilisation occurs, and then transfer of the embryo to the tube when the environment for the embryo may be better than the laboratory.

Most patients suitable for PROST (ZIFT) or TEST are also suitable for GIFT. Exceptions are after microinjection of sperm into the egg where IVF is obligatory to determine fertilisation, or where sperm is aspirated from a blockage in the male genital tract and IVF attempted with a small quantity of sperm of variable quality.

If GIFT fails on several occasions and there have been no excess eggs to check for fertilisation by IVF, the possibility of barriers to fertilisation in the sperm or eggs exists. IVF should be pursued on one occasion to check that fertilisation is possible. If fertilisation is proven, it is best to persist with GIFT because of its higher success rate.

A small number of patients have repeated failed fertilisations. These patients should be checked for sperm antibodies in sperm or female plasma and for anti-lupus or anti-cardiolipin antibodies in the female that may cause infertility. Chromosome studies in male and female plasma, sperm binding to stored eggs, and, if the opportunity arises, study of chromosomes in a crop of eggs produced by IVF should also be carried out. Microinjection of sperm into eggs is an option which may overcome barriers to fertilisation at the zona (shell) of the egg. In older women, failed fertilisation is most likely due to poor egg quality and they may wish to consider using donor eggs from a younger woman.

Donor egg

Less than a decade ago, women who suffered premature menopause, those who had their ovaries surgically removed or those undergoing chemotherapy treatment had no hope of having a family.

Today, thanks to the donor egg program, that has changed. Women who fail to produce good quality eggs for IVF can also use donor eggs.

Obviously it is more difficult to get women to donate eggs than for men to donate sperm because women actually have to undergo an IVF process. For this reason, the women who donate eggs are motivated and keen to help.

More than half the eggs used in the donor egg program come from known donors such as a close relative or friend. In Victoria, it is legal to use both known and unknown donors.

Unknown donors are usually women who themselves are undergoing IVF who have decided to donate their "excess" eggs.

The pregnant woman is considered the legal mother and the donor has no legal responsibility to the child, nor has the child any claim on the donor (this applies to both egg and sperm donors).

Donor eggs are also a means of allowing older women to have a healthy child. Women over 40 have reduced fertility and those who are lucky enough to get pregnant have a high risk of miscarriage.

Older women also face a higher risk of foetal deformity including Downs Syndrome, so the option of using an egg donated by a younger woman allays many fears.

Known donors have a higher success rate because they give all their eggs to one recipient. Many unknown donors, as mentioned, are on IVF programs themselves and can therefore give only their 'leftovers' which are in excess of their own needs.

The follow up of families with children from donor eggs has, up to date, shown no problems. The known donors may act as a friend or 'aunty' to the child, or never see the child. It is important for the donor and recipient to have a satisfactory relationship.

In recent months, we have appealed for egg donors. Obviously, those women with a 'known' donor overcome the problem of waiting for donor eggs to become available.

Ideally, a donor should be aged between 25 to 35 years and have already proven herself by having children of her own. She would usually have finished her own family and be in a stable relationship.

Strict counselling is compulsory for both the donor and recipient and their partners.

This is one of the most wonderful gifts one woman can give another and we are hoping to attract increasing numbers of donors to reduce the current 12-month waiting list for unknown donors.

Freezing

An IVF treatment may be used to produce frozen embryos and not proceed with fresh embryo transfer. This is done for women with severe acute illnesses requiring urgent treatment, such as leukemia or cancer. The treatment may render the woman sterile by damaging the ovaries. When treatment is successful the frozen embryos can be transferred back to the patient at a later date, the pregnancy being supported artificially by hormones in the first weeks of pregnancy.

Some clinics have frozen all embryos and put them back in a natural cycle 1 or 2 months later. Implantation may not be so effective in the treatment cycle because of the effect of the stimulation on the lining of the uterus. However freezing itself may harm embryos as only 70 per cent survive the process. The gains from transferring the frozen embryos in a natural cycle may not be sufficient to counter the disadvantage of freezing and thawing embryos, so most clinics only freeze excess embryos.

4
COMMON QUESTIONS ABOUT IVF

What test do I need before starting IVF?

One blood test for women detects rubella, hepatitis B, HIV (AIDS) virus and sperm antibodies.
　The male has a blood test for hepatitis B and HIV (AIDS) virus antibodies. Also two semen tests are done, including a check for sperm antibodies and infection.

Does my husband need a semen analysis before starting IVF?

Yes, at least one semen analysis should be performed at the Infertility Medical Centre's laboratory prior to treatment. These analyses include tests for sperm antibodies in the semen and check for possible infection that may affect fertilisation.

Do all couples need counselling?

Yes, it is a legal requirement. Under Victorian legislation, all potential IVF couples must attend a counselling session prior to treatment. This can be arranged on an individual basis and is regarded as an information giving session.

Is there a waiting list after we have been accepted?

Yes, but that is decreasing all the time. Most couples can begin treatment within three to four months.

What are my chances of achieving a pregnancy?

Of every 100 new patients starting on the IVF program, 85 will get as far as egg pick-up; 75 will make it to embryo transfer; 15 will actually achieve a pregnancy and 10 will achieve a live birth.

The comparable figures for GIFT, 85 as far as egg pick-up; 30 achieve a pregnancy and 20 will achieve a live birth.

What about multiple pregnancy?

There is a risk of multiple pregnancy. If, for example, you have three embryos transferred and a pregnancy is achieved, 85 per cent of the pregnancies will be single, 14 per cent will result in a twin pregnancy and 1 per cent of the pregnancies will be triplet pregnancies. We have reduced the risk of triplets by reducing the number of eggs replaced in GIFT and embryos replaced in IVF.

What decisions do we need to make at the start of each treatment cycle?

If the husband has no or insufficient sperm, donor sperm may be used for IVF and GIFT. Occasionally, if the husband's sperm is of borderline quality, both donor and husband sperm may be used to inseminate separate eggs. You must choose how many eggs you want to be inseminated with donor sperm and how many with your husband's sperm.

You may have to decide what to do with eggs in excess of your requirements. Your choices are to donate to research and/or another patient, donate to research only, donate to another patient only or to discard the excess eggs. We have a donor egg program in which patients who cannot produce eggs of their own, rely on donor eggs.

How many embryos can I have transferred?

You are allowed a maximum of three but the choice of how many you wish transferred must be made by you and your husband. When making that decision, remember that the chance of pregnancy increases with the number of embryos transferred. The risk of multiple pregnancy also increases with an increasing number of embryos transferred.

We understand that it is difficult to come to a final decision before you are informed as to the number and quality of your embryos which occurs at the time of embryo transfer.

However, you and your husband should have discussed the alternatives and you will be required to sign a consent form at the start of the cycle stating the maximum number of embryos you wish to be transferred.

Your final decision will be made at the time of embryo transfer with information from the clinician and scientist. If you are older, more embryos are transferred as the chance of pregnancy is lower and multiple pregnancy very uncommon.

Those patients using the GIFT technique are advised to transfer between two and three eggs with sperm into your fallopian tubes. This is based on your age and quality of eggs collected. If you are over 40 years, more than three eggs can be transferred. If the sperm quality is low you can also use up to six eggs.

What if I don't want to have any embryos frozen?

If you don't wish to have embryos frozen, all eggs are picked up but only the best three are inseminated. The remaining eggs can be donated to another patient, research or discarded.

Victorian legislation prevents us from inseminating all eggs, selecting the best three or four for embryo transfer and discarding the remainder as this amounts to creating embryos without the intention of using them in a fertilisation procedure.

What happens to the frozen embryos in the event of death or divorce?

You must decide if the frozen embryos are to be donated to research, donated to another patient or disposed of before you start your treatment cycle. If one partner wishes to use the embryos after divorce, court application may be necessary.

Do we need private cover?

The program is privately run and the total cost is relatively high, so it is advisable that most couples have private health cover.

Remember, IVF is treated as a pre-existing condition by the health funds so to be eligible from a fund, patients must have been members for at least 12 months.

Women can take out a Singles cover, if only the woman is being treated. However, you may run into difficulties should you become pregnant and want your pregnancy privately insured. This is something you should discuss with your Health Fund.

What treatments are covered by health insurance?

In general, IVF tests and treatments are covered by Government Rebates and health insurance and you need only pay a small percentage of the actual cost. But there are some items for which there is no rebate.

Some items are only covered by particular schedules but there is a lot of variation so it is best if you discuss this with your own health fund.

When scheduled fees are charged, Medicare covers 85 per cent of the costs of medical consultations, laboratory tests and ultrasound scans. There is a maximum "gap" with the Medicare Schedule so once you have paid $150 yourself, you should inform Medicare as all benefits over and above this amount are 100 per cent.

What about in-patient procedures?

These are covered by Medicare at the rate of 75 per cent of schedule fee and private health insurance can be taken out to cover this gap. The majority of charges from IMC and its associated medical staff are charged at, or close to, schedule fee. Private hospital insurance covers some or all of the costs of the hospital bed and the operating fee.

What are the out of pocket costs for a privately insured patient?

Currently, the cost for a privately insured patient undergoing a standard IVF/GIFT/TEST cycle is $250 to $500; this includes embryo freezing costs. For those overseas couples with no Medicare insurance the cost is $3,500 per cycle.

How long can we have embryos frozen?

Long term storage of frozen embryos is possible but not encouraged. If frozen embryos are stored for longer than two years, the couple may be interviewed by their doctor.
 Embryo storage longer than five years requires specific reasons to be registered with the Attorney General's Department. Storage for more than three months attracts a fee.

When would we look at a frozen embryo cycle?

If vaginal bleeding makes transfer of the fresh embryo(s) undesirable or if a medical condition contra-indicates the transfer of fresh embryos, embryos can be frozen for later use.
 If pregnancy has not resulted from a fresh embryo transfer, frozen embryo thawing and transfer is recommended during one of the following menstrual cycles.

How many embryos should you have frozen for the next attempt?

If only one embryo is frozen from the original cycle, it is recommended that further IVF cycles are undertaken in order to have at least two or three embryos frozen for subsequent thawing and transfer cycle. This increases the chances of pregnancy.
 Transfer of a single frozen has a success rate of about 9 per cent, transfer of two frozen embryos a success rate of 18 per cent.

Common Questions about In Vitro Fertilisation

What are the chances of the embryos surviving the thawing procedure?

Approximately three quarters survive in a condition which is suitable for transfer.

When do I find out if I am pregnant?

A blood test is carried out at day 28 and the result of the pregnancy test will be given to you by the clinic.

What about my next treatment?

The centre will send you a letter suggesting a plan for your next treatment. If you agree with this proposal you need not see your clinician.
 Regardless of the outcome of a treatment cycle, you will also be offered an appointment with your IVF clinician a couple of weeks after the end of the cycle. If you are not pregnant, this is a chance to review the treatment cycle and to discuss plans for future cycles should you wish.
 If you are pregnant, the clinician needs to plan your follow-up over the next couple of months.

When do I contact the clinic to start treatment?

Phone the centre well before the expected time of your proposed treatment cycle.

When do I see my own doctor?

You see your own doctor before you start your treatment to finalise arrangements for treatment. The Centre will plan further treatments and write to you after each treatment. You can also see your own doctor after each treatment if you wish further discussion.

What does a single treatment involve?

On average you have 8-9 injections, two blood collections and ultrasound pictures, 3 visits to the clinic (before the period, day 8 and 10), a day in hospital having the eggs picked up under anaesthesia or sedation, and a return visit 2 days later to have the embryos transferred usually without drugs or anaesthesia. GIFT patients have the eggs picked up and transferred with the sperm on the same day. Injections can be given at home or at a local clinic.

THE IN VITRO FERTILIZATION TECHNIQUE

The IVF technique is used primarily to treat infertility. A mature egg (oocyte) is collected from the woman's ovary and fertilized with the husband's sperm.

The resulting embryo is then cultured in an incubator until the four to eight cell stage of development.

The embryo is then transferred to the woman's uterus where its development continues in the normal manner.

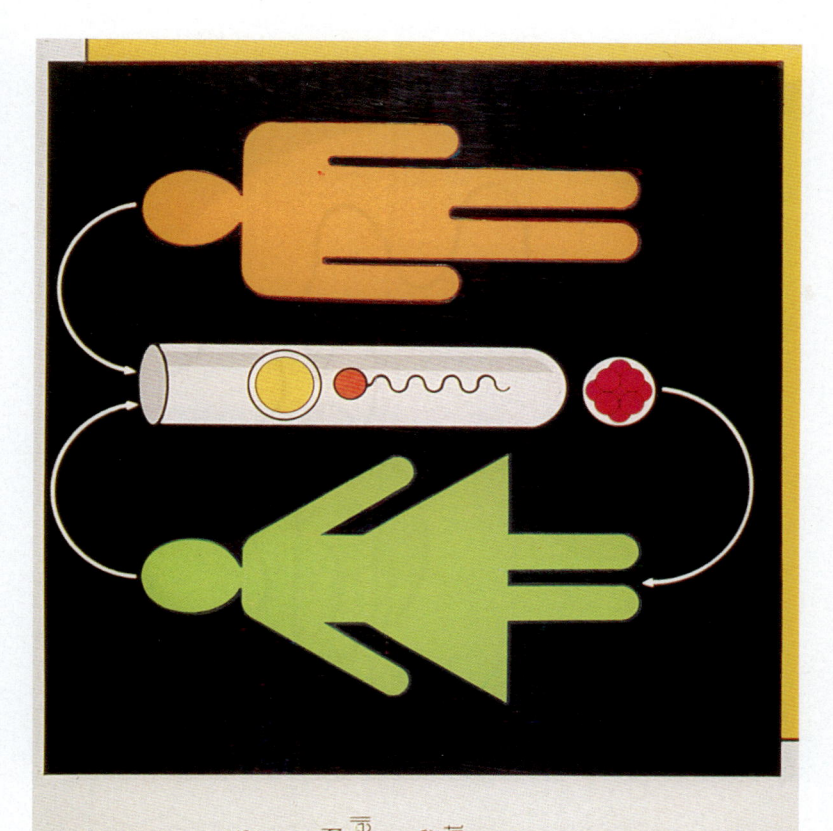

MALE FACTOR GROUP

As mentioned previously, when the number of sperm, the number of swimming sperm or the number of normal sperm is below normal, special care has to be taken in preparing the sperm for IVF. This is done by the IMC Male Factor group. Special techniques for preparing the sperm allow subnormal sperm to be used for IVF. While IVF was originally designed for the treatment of female factor infertility, IVF has now become the most successful treatment for male factor infertility. The main question that is asked about male factor infertility is "What causes it?". Unfortunately, while we know of many causes of reduced sperm quality, it is very difficult to say what caused the problem in an individual. However, it is known that excess heat (eg. saunas), sexually transmitted diseases, some drugs and some heavy metals can cause a reduction in sperm quality.

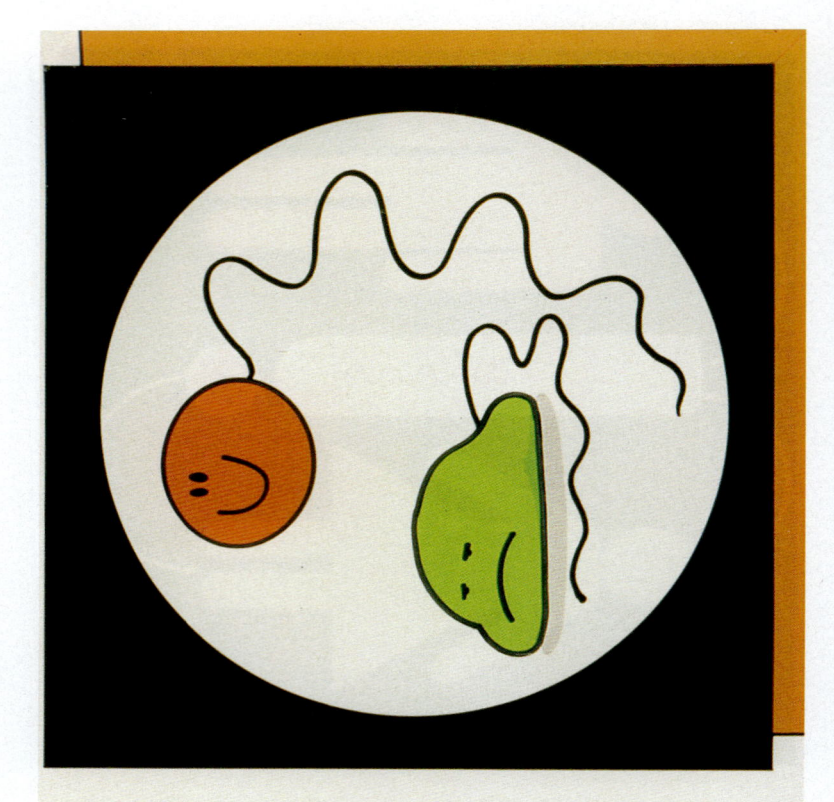

Donor

Fertilization

Recipient — Example of abnormal ovaries — Hormone Stimulation

The donated egg is fertilized with the recipients husband's sperm and then transferred to her uterus.

The uterus is artificially stimulated with oestrogen and progesterone to condition it ready for pregnancy before the embryo is transferred to the uterus.

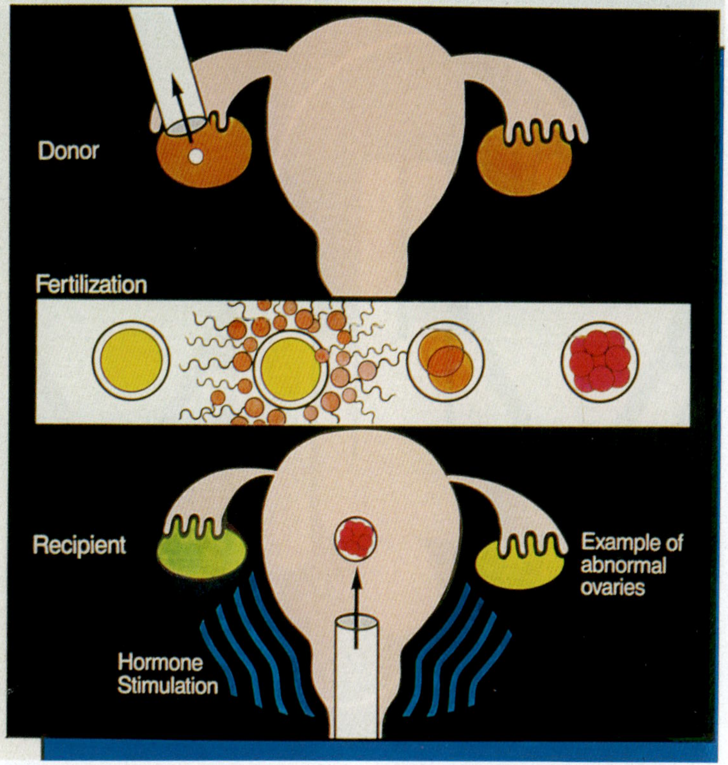

THE DONOR EGG PROJECT

If a woman's ovaries are absent, non-functioning or if she carries an abnormal gene, a donated egg can be used.

Couples can choose whether they would like to have a known or unknown donor. Sperm from the recipients husband is used to fertilize the donated egg.

In cases where the ovaries are absent or non-functioning, hormone replacement therapy is needed.

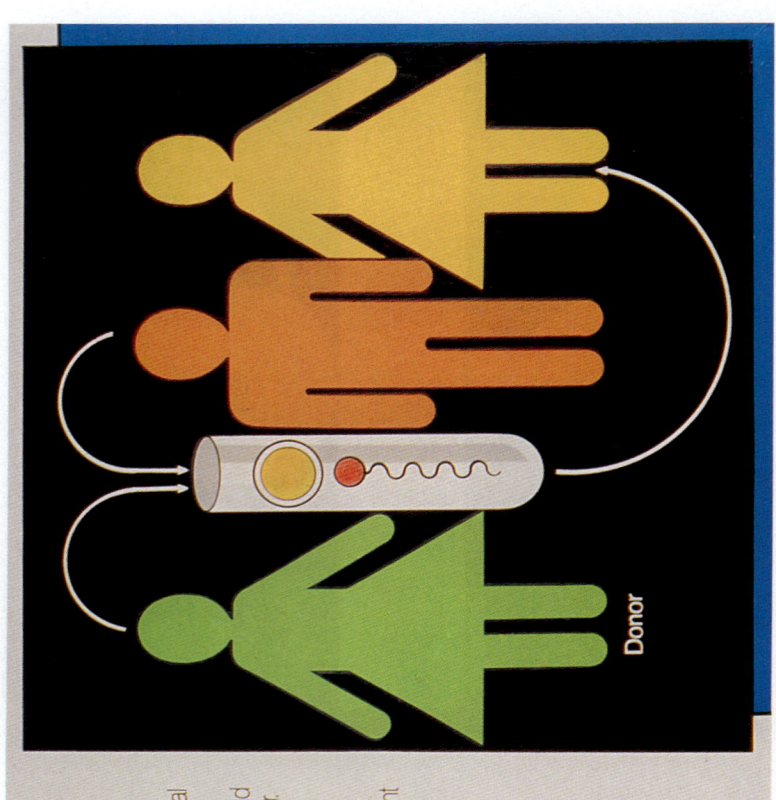

Donor

SPERM & IVF

Many people think that the sperm can just be added to the egg in IVF. This is not the case, as the seminal fluid (the fluid which carries the sperm) will not only stop fertilization from occurring, but will also kill the egg. To prepare the sperm for IVF, the semen sample is washed in the same media that the egg is kept in. The sperm are then placed in a test-tube and fresh media placed on top of them. The sperm then swim up into the fresh media and, after about 30 minutes, the fresh media containing the sperm is removed. It is this fresh media containing motile sperm that is added to the egg. Contrary to the opinion that "it only takes one", at least 50,000 swimming sperm have to be added to each egg. Of course, only one sperm penetrates the egg.

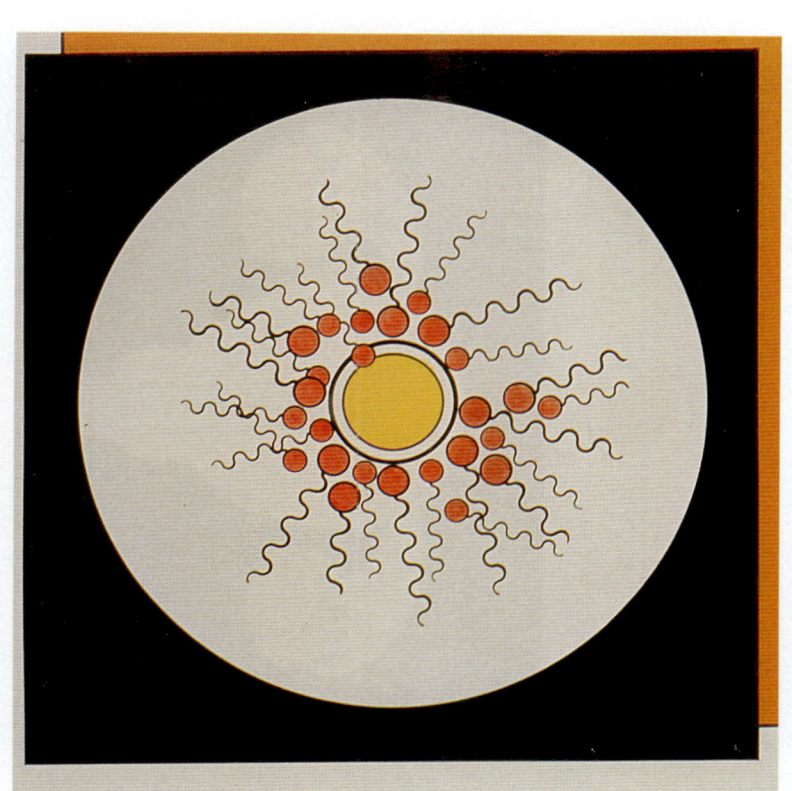

Egg Culture and Fertilization

Prepared sperm are placed with the individual eggs to encourage fertilization. The process of cell division begins.

Embryo Transfer

The developing embryo is inserted back into the uterus using a fine Teflon catheter.

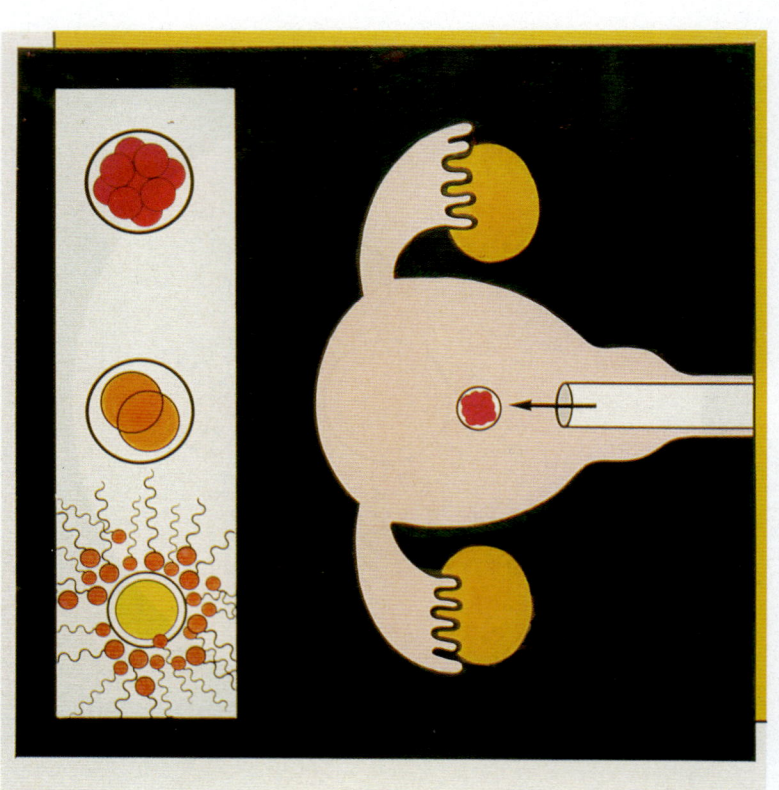

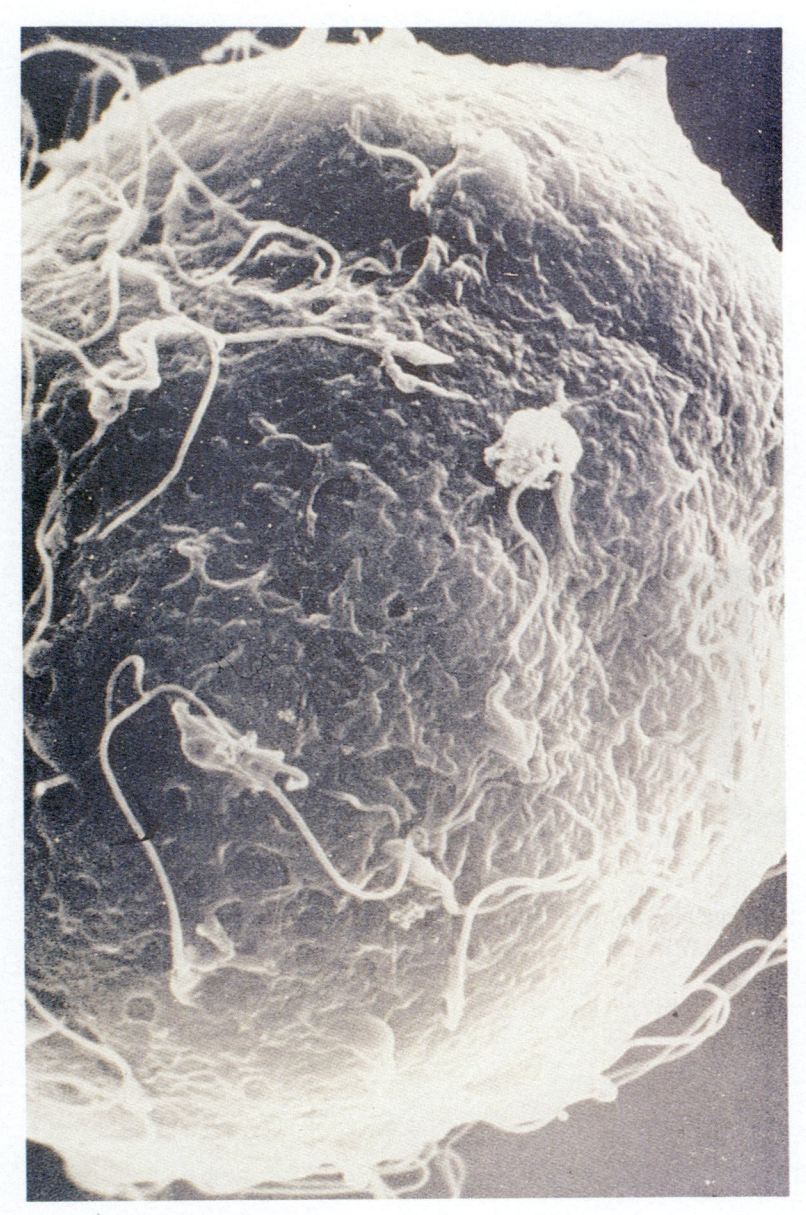

Sperm penetrating egg

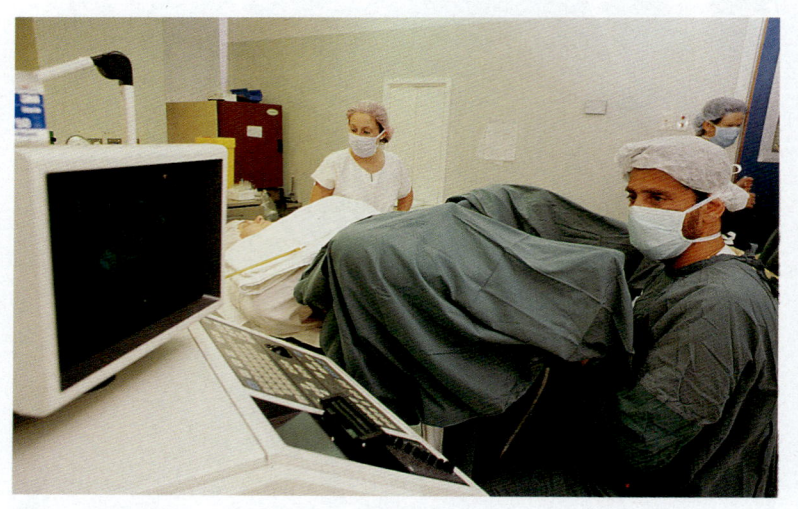

The egg pick-up is by vaginal ultrasound or laparoscopy.

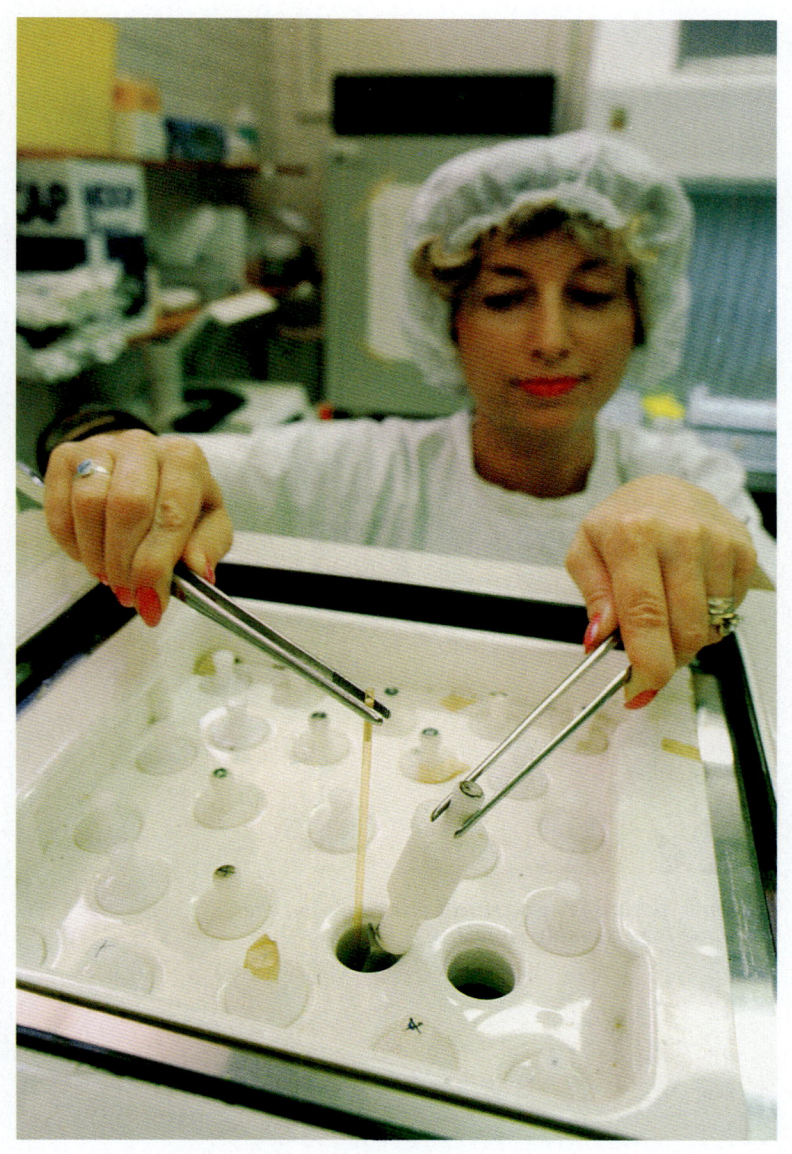

Laboratory assistant shows embryos being frozen for storage. This procedure has gradually improved over the years.

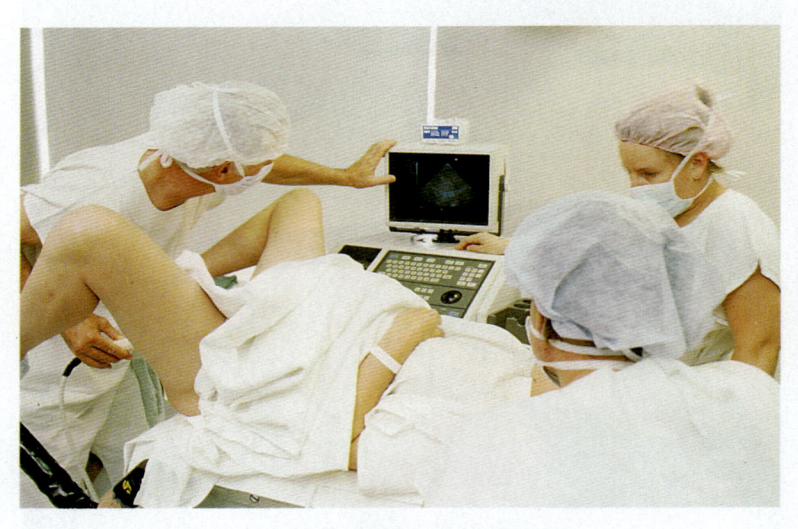

The embryo transfer is a critical procedure but the technique is reasonably simple.

Gamete
Intra
Fallopian
Transfer

IVF Australia

PERCENT OF MULTIPLE BIRTHS
IVF AUSTRALIA PROGRAMS
Consolidated

Number of Embryos Transferred	Singletons	Twins	Triplets	Quads
1	100%	0%	0%	0%
2	92%	8%	0%	0%
3	75%	25%	0%	0%
4	60%	30%	9%	0%

IVF Australia

5
TELLING IT LIKE IT IS

One of the best ways to explain IVF, its emotional and physical costs and what the patients think about the procedures is to talk to couples involved.

In this chapter we have asked three patients to talk about their own experiences. They talk about their expectations, their disappointments and their future.

There are success stories as well as those who have not succeeded—yet!

SUSAN AND GERARD'S STORY (IVF)

Susan and Gerard consider themselves lucky. They have three children thanks to the In-Vitro Fertilisation program. But Susan is the first to admit it wasn't easy. This is their story.

We have been married for ten years and started trying to conceive about two years after we married. When things didn't happen as we had expected, I had a laparoscopy which confirmed my tubes were blocked which was caused through an infection from an IUD.

I had surgery to try and correct the damage to my tubes but this was not successful as too much damage had already been done. The laparoscopy showed that both tubes were totally blocked and it seemed, at the time, that we would never conceive. We were devastated.

That was in 1982. We were told it might be a good idea if we put our names down on the IVF waiting list. We had heard a little of the program but thought it was something that would happen in the future—most likely too far in the future to be of help to us.

I read what I could find about the program and put my name down on the waiting list. To be honest though, I never really thought I would hear any more about it so we both decided to just get on with our lives.

Then about 12 months later I received a letter that was to change our lives.

The letter told us we had been accepted on the program and could come in for counselling. We couldn't believe it! We never thought it would happen in time for us.

We were a little apprehensive, as IVF was still in its early stages, but as we had no alternatives we decided to go ahead. How lucky that we did! On my first cycle I had three eggs implanted and fell pregnant immediately.

How did I feel to hear the news that I was pregnant? Over the moon, ecstatic, elated, happy. And yes, to be honest, I guess a little frightened at first. People have often asked me did I find the program painful, did I find it intrusive? To be honest I never found the daily blood tests and injections painful. I handled them OK. I was probably luckier than some because we decided that it would be best for me to give up work before starting the program so although the waiting for blood tests and injections was at times annoying, I never had that anxiety about being late for work.

Also, I think we were both so excited about being involved with the program at such an early stage. I don't think either of us expected our first attempt to be successful. We were prepared to have several attempts and I believe that attitude helped to keep us calm and relaxed about the whole thing.

I also got myself as healthy and fit as possible beforehand which I believe is essential.

Probably the hardest part of the cycle was ringing up for the pregnancy results. You are so nervous before you dial the number and then you just pray the answer will be 'positive'. When I heard that I was indeed pregnant, I can't describe how I felt. It was just so unbelievable.

Naturally you have some fears and concerns. I didn't tell many people—other than close family members—that we had conceived using IVF. It took me about a year after my daughter was born to feel confident enough to tell people how she was conceived. By then I was just so proud of her that I wanted everyone to know she was an IVF baby.

After her birth I knew that we would go through the program again because we both wanted another child. Again, I think I went with the right attitude because if it failed this time, at least we had our daughter and we knew how lucky we were anyway.

I wanted to spend at least two years with my daughter before starting the program again, and that's what we did.

But the second time around it took us six cycles to achieve another pregnancy. I am not sure what I expected the second time around. I was fairly relaxed about it all and because I had already been through once, I was not apprehensive about the treatment and I knew what to expect.

I think it had improved because there was an effort to make life as easy as possible for everyone concerned. Injections, for example, are now given by the husbands and Gerard was great about that. He did a first aid course and learnt how to administer the injection which made life a lot easier, especially with a toddler to think about.

As each cycle failed I would always say to myself: 'At least we are lucky enough to have a child', but I must admit that it is devastating to be told you are not pregnant after you have pinned all your hopes on this cycle.

It would take me two months to get over that news, another two months to forget all about IVF and a further two months to get myself keyed up for another attempt.

People ask what is the most difficult part of IVF and I still say it is ringing up for your pregnancy result. I hated that. You would dial the number, tell them who was calling and then take a deep breath and wait for a yes or no.

If it was no, you would get off the phone as quickly as possible, have a good cry and then try to come to terms with the news as quickly as you could. I found that I could cope better if I sat down and tried to work out what went wrong and how could we do better the next time.

For six weeks after the result I would be really depressed until I went to see my clinician who would then say: "Well it didn't work this time but next time we will do this or try that". Then

I would walk out of his office smiling and start preparing for the next attempt. He was wonderful, very supportive and full of encouragement and it was him who boosted my spirits and encouraged me to try another attempt.

We went through that five times! When we started the sixth attempt we both agreed it would be our last and we meant it. I think we both had had enough and it becomes very difficult to keep thinking positive when you have been through five attempts unsuccessfully. Again I went through the process of talking to my doctor about what may have gone wrong the last time, where we could make changes for a better attempt this time.

He agreed to let me start taking Clomid on day six because I had a lengthy cycle. I had three eggs implanted and then at last we got the news we had so desperately waited for. I was pregnant again.

The next exciting thing was to have a scan to see how many babies we would have.

Twins! Our beautiful baby boys were born by Caesarean section.

When we first married and discussed, like most young couples, our hopes for a family, we decided we would like three children. Now, thanks to our wonderful doctor and the IVF we have the family we wanted.

People talk about the cost involved, the financial strain. Yes, it is difficult and there are many hidden costs we had not expected and which are not covered by Medicare. The fact that I left work as soon as I started on the program made it even more difficult financially.

But when everything is said and done, the result for us has been fantastic. Beyond our wildest dreams. So despite the cost, the medication, the injections, the blood tests, the fear and the anxiety, I would go through it all again.

My advice is to have a positive attitude and don't expect to succeed immediately. Give yourself a goal. Say you are prepared to go through a cycle five or six, eight, ten times! And be prepared for the disappointment. But in the end, IVF gives us a chance to have the family that not too many years ago would have been an impossible dream.

SUE AND JOHN'S STORY (DONOR EGG)

Sue and John O'Brien consider themselves very fortunate. They have a beautiful baby son and hope to have another child soon.

For Sue who suffered a chronic kidney condition as a child, having a family of her own is something she never thought possible.

"When I was 18 I was put on drugs to treat my kidney condition," she said. "My ovaries were severely damaged and I actually went through menopause when I was 22 years old."

The Melbourne woman said she was devastated to experience 'the change of life' just 12 months after she married her husband John. "At first I didn't know what menopause meant,"she said.

"I was experiencing hot flushes and then my periods stopped all together and we were told we could never hope to have children."

Sue and John were in their early 20s, newly married and had to come to terms with a life without children.

"I guess because of my kidney condition, we were prepared in a way," Sue said. "But when someone actually says it out loud, tells you you can't have a baby, that's still devastating."

For more than a decade, the couple got on with their lives.

Then in 1986, Sue overheard a radio show discussing the IVF program and donor eggs.

"I went straight to my doctor to ask about this program and was referred to an IVF specialist immediately," Sue said.

"It was exciting to think that just maybe there was still a chance for us to have a family."

"The specialist was surprised to learn that I had not been put on Hormone Replacement Therapy when I went through menopause 13 years earlier.

"That made me angry to think that this was available and nobody had bothered to tell me."

Sue was immediately placed on oestrogen and had to undergo a kidney biopsy before being admitted to the IVF program.

"I could understand why I had to have a biopsy. Obviously the doctors wanted to make sure I could carry a baby if I was lucky enough to get pregnant."

Sue said it was difficult waiting for the results of the biopsy. "I kept thinking that finally something was available to help me become a mother and maybe my kidneys would not hold up to a pregnancy."

She need not have worried. The biopsy was fine and Sue joined a waiting list for the donor egg program.

She was 34 years old and was told that if she could find her own donor, she could join the program immediately.

"Obviously if you have someone ready to donate eggs for you, it is much better. The waiting list for donor eggs is about 18 months."

Sue and John had discussed their plight with a friend sometime before. She said that if she could help at any time, give her a call.

"When I rang and asked if she would donate an egg, my friend didn't have to think twice. She said she would be happy to do it."

Donating an egg meant Sue's girlfriend had to go through an IVF cycle to have the eggs collected. The first time around, five eggs were collected. Three were placed in Sue's uterus. Two were frozen.

"I was so excited," Sue said. "I kept thinking how wonderful it was to have five eggs."

But Sue received a letter a week before she was to have her pregnancy test telling her the two eggs were not suitable for freezing.

"I thought well if those two were no good, the three that had been placed in me would be no good either. I was very disappointed."

The results of Sue's first pregnancy test confirmed her fears. It was negative.

When her friend learned the news, she offered to donate eggs again.

"She was fantastic, very supportive and encouraging," Sue said. "So four months later, we went through the process again."

This time four eggs were collected and placed in Sue. Sue did become pregnant but unfortunately the pregnancy only lasted five days.

"I was terribly upset, naturally, but I knew that at least I could get pregnant. There was some hope."

Sue didn't want to ask her girlfriend to donate eggs again and decided to take her chances with the donor egg waiting list.

"Finally my name came to the top of the unknown donor list and in November, 1987, I was ready to have another go."

Sue was to receive five eggs, but she was only at day two of her cycle and her uterus was not ready to receive the eggs. Three of the eggs available were fertilised and one was frozen. But unfortunately a pregnancy did not result.

Finally in October, 1988, Sue was ready to try another unknown donor egg cycle.

Two eggs were placed in her and the O'Briens finally heard the news they had been waiting to hear for so many years—Sue was pregnant with a viable pregnancy.

"We still had our nervous moments. I had to have a blood test every Friday until I was 13 weeks to check my hormone levels. I used to dread those days," Sue laughed.

At 28 weeks she experienced some spotting but Sue enjoyed a relatively normal pregnancy until the last few months.

"My son was born four weeks early and I had to spend the last three weeks of the pregnancy in hospital so they could keep an eye on my kidneys," she said.

"People often ask if Timothy feels like my own son because he is the result of a donor egg. I carried him in a normal pregnancy, gave birth to him and nurtured him. He is our beautiful son and we love him."

Sue and John plan to try the unknown donor program again. "There is still an 18-month waiting list because people are still unaware of this program. It is difficult to attract egg donors and that is why there is such a long waiting list," she said.

"But it is worth the wait," she smiles.

MARY'S STORY (GIFT)

'Mary' joined the IVF program in 1987 after suffering the miscarriage of twins, eight weeks into her first pregnancy.

I was 40 and although we hadn't been trying for a family for all that long, I realised both my husband and I were getting older.

I became pregnant with the twins naturally, so never really considered there could be a problem with my fertility.

But a friend suggested that 'at our age' we really should be under the best possible care and, in my opinion, the best person was Carl Wood.

After coming out of hospital to see him after the miscarriage, I rang up and made an appointment three days later.

Initially I thought he was going to think I was neurotic. Straight out of hospital and making an appointment to see a fertility specialist!

But he didn't of course. After my first consultation I knew I had at last found someone I could relate to.

I underwent hormone tests which revealed a high prolactin level. A course of drugs was prescribed to lower that level and my hopes were high for another pregnancy.

The following month, not pregnant, more tests revealed I had hostile mucous and it was suggested I try Intrauterine Insemination using my husband's sperm.

I think I had about six attempts at IUI but I was never successful in getting pregnant. I didn't see this as a wasted effort though because it offered a great transition to undertaking IVF. It helped me to understand and appreciate what would be involved, such as the early morning blood tests, ultrasound scans and basically getting into a routine.

By the end of 1988 I was started on delayed GIFT (a procedure where the eggs are collected in the morning and returned via laparoscopy with the husband's sperm that afternoon into the top of the fallopian tubes).

To prepare ourselves for that procedure, my husband and I made sure that we had all the necessary tests done before our name came to the top of the list so that when I received notification that we could start the program, we would have no delays.

The first month I ovulated before I got to theatre. The clinicians were able to catch one egg. This was transferred back into the tube later that day. However, we knew the success rate with only one egg was minimal. The negative pregnancy test confirmed this 14 days later.

Like all patients, my first attempt had to be on Clomid and by the second treatment I was eligible to try Buserelin. However, for some unknown reason my follicles didn't develop satisfactorily and therefore this program cycle was cancelled. I know some couples get angry and upset when they are called off the program but the way I look at it, I have faith in the clinicians.

Rather than make you go through the ordeal of anaesthetics and surgery they are honest and tell you straight out that there is not much hope. I admire that.

The third attempt I went to theatre and had six eggs picked up. I had the six transferred using the delayed GIFT procedure.

That meant I underwent two anaesthetics in one day. The first in the morning to retrieve the eggs and the second that afternoon when they were put back using laparoscopy.

It is amazing what you will put yourself through. You can program yourself to endure extreme stress in order to achieve your goal. I was delighted when we were told I was pregnant that cycle. We had six eggs put back and were expecting a multiple pregnancy but were still delighted with a single pregnancy.

We had the usual early scan which showed this tiny sac with a fluttering heartbeat and it seemed everything was going to plan.

Another scan at 12 weeks was remarkable. Legs, arms, heartbeat, everything was there.

That scan was a lengthy procedure because the specialist had to monitor everything carefully. Afterwards, we asked if all was well. The specialist appeared a little uncomfortable and said there was a slight problem.

Our hearts sank. The slight problem he referred to was a thin hairline membrane stretching from the base of the baby's head down its back.

The specialist said it could be a chromosomal problem and because of my age, that could indicate Downs or Turner Syndrome. We were devastated.

When we first learnt of the pregnancy, we decided against an amniocentesis test because of the risk factor.

Now, we really had no choice. Four weeks later we underwent the test.

The next day I started losing fluid and rang my doctor to tell him I had lost about 4 tablespoons of fluid.

By 9 am we were sitting in his office and when he started a pelvic examination, more fluid gushed out. He said the membrane had ruptured and I would be in labour within a few hours.

I was put in hospital and waited for the worst. But the contractions never started and a week later another scan showed the fluid had replaced itself and that the membrane had healed. Incredibly, the baby was still alive but we still had one last hurdle. We had to wait for the test results.

On the day I was supposed to return to work, we were told the news that our much-wanted baby had Downs Syndrome.

We were devastated and decided to go ahead with a termination.

I am a practising Catholic so it was a difficult decision for me to make. But unfortunately, most Down Syndrome babies are severely retarded and I could not bring a baby into the world to suffer.

The termination was traumatic. Luckily my doctor said he would leave the decision up to me regarding pain killers and drugs.

I went into hospital on Saturday morning. The birth was induced over a twelve hour period. At 9.30 that night contractions started with the birth at 3.20am the next day.

I was uptight right throughout the procedure. I had never experienced childbirth before and didn't know what to expect— of course the mind plays havoc upon one so naive.

Prior to entering hospital, I requested permission for a relaxation therapist to be present. He helped me throughout the termination with hypnotherapy.

Finally, after a combination of pain killers, epidural and hypno- therapy, our baby was born. It was a boy.

I didn't want to know what sex the baby was. Even when I had the scan and amnio test, I asked not to be told because I didn't want to bond with the baby.

After he was born, the afterbirth wouldn't come away and my doctor was called in. I told him I didn't feel up to going through a curette and he agreed to let me go home to rest. It was suggested that I wait at least 12 months before trying again. But I was determined to try for a baby as soon as possible.

We decided I should have a scan to make sure the uterus had recovered from the termination and it was discovered that afterbirth was still present. I had to undergo a curette which meant a further wait of two months before I could start another cycle.

Since the termination, I have been back on the program four times to date. The first two attempts were cancelled prior to theatre due to poor follicle growth.

On my third attempt, I was "Down Regulated" resulting in a six egg pick up and six egg transfer, however, a pregnancy did not occur—my husband's sperm abnormality rating had increased dramatically, thus reducing our chances for fertilisation.

We were then advised to:
    i) see an endocrinologist;
    ii) try "Tubal Embryo Stage Transfer" (T.E.S.T.) in future;

Our appointment with the endocrinologist was most informative. It was brought to our attention during this meeting that there could be a correlation between my husband's sperm abnormality and a medically prescribed drug he had been taking for an arthritic-related condition.

At this stage I was back on the program. In February 1991, I had four eggs collected, two of which fertilised. One stopped cleaving prior to theatre therefore only one embryo was transferred. Again, because of my age, the success rate with one embryo is minimal. Pregnancy did not result, but hopefully we'll have better luck next time.

Since mid-January, my husband has been withdrawn from all forms of medication. We are optimistic that the next sperm analysis will show a marked improvement. I personally hope to be back in theatre by mid-April and am praying that the next program will succeed.

People may wonder why you put yourself through all of this, well IVF is our only answer. When we discovered that we had a fertility problem, we looked at adoption and were told we were too old.

So then we considered inter-country adoption only to learn the Minister had closed the books and those books are still closed.

We have tried every approach and IVF is the only answer for us.

Because of my age, and the subsequent quality of my eggs, we have been advised to seriously consider the Donor Egg program. We have registered for this and will have the option to start later this year.

I have been lobbying the Government to change the laws governing embryo biopsy because I have to believe that something positive will come out of the termination I had to endure.

If embryo biopsy was endorsed, I wouldn't have to go through the trauma of carrying a child only to find out it has Downs Syndrome. I believe the Government should allow testing for any woman over 37, as well as those known to be carriers of genetic diseases. No one should be subjected to the suffering, disappointment and heartbreak we have been made to endure.

One way or another, my husband and I hope to have a child. How long will I keep going? Until the clinicians close the doors on us!

I want to be able to say well we did everything we possibly could. Having a child is that important to us.

SUPPORT GROUPS

Groups such as IVF Friends provide an invaluable support system both to those on the program and to IMC itself. IVF Friends has been helpful in making constructive critisisms to IMC about how to improve patient care.

IVF Friends was formed in 1980 by couples taking part in the Monash University IVF Program at the Queen Victoria Medical Centre in Melbourne.

It now boasts a membership Australia-wide of more than 1000 couples who come from a wide range of religious and ethnic backgrounds representing varying philosophical and moral viewpoints.

The executive committee says that by remaining non-sectarian and non-political, the group can devote its resource to the issues relating to infertility, in particular IVF, and to the well-being of couples on the program or waiting to join it.

The aims of the group include:
- To provide moral support for members through the creation of a supportive environment and the development of new friendships.
- To assist members to understand the in vitro fertilisation embryo transplant techniques as well as other forms of treatment for infertility.
- To raise money for the in vitro fertilisation program, primarily to assist in the purchase of medical equipment to be used in the program.
- To undertake any other voluntary work which IVF Friends' members may from time to time see fit.

The IVF team recognises the role being played by IVF Friends and we encourage and co-operate in the two-way flow of ideas and information between patients and doctors.

At the same time, IVF Friends functions autonomously and its major concern is to represent its members' interests. The group's secretary said it was important to stress that IVF Friends is a separate entity from the Infertility Medical Centre and that all correspondence is confidential.

Members receive a monthly newsletter which keeps them up to date with new technologies, changes in treatment procedures and information about Team members, details of relevant literature and an update of what is appearing in the media generally about infertility and IVF.

Through regular meetings with the Team, the group is able to pass on thoughts from patients (anonymously, of course!) and to receive feedback about IVF routines, techniques and personnel which is of interest to those on the program.

The newsletter also includes a listing of the current members of the executive committee and members are welcome to contact any members of this committee directly.

General meetings for all members are held on the last Tuesday of every second month at 7.30pm at Epworth Hospital, 34 Erin Street, Richmond, Victoria. Often guest speakers attend to discuss issues relating to infertility and IVF treatments and the related physical and psychological effects remedies.

The wish for privacy is treated with respect and membership rolls are kept confidential.

Remember, often talking with someone who has been through the program helps reduce anxiety about some aspects of treatment. If requested, a member of the group will even visit the IVF ward at Epworth Hospital to chat with patients and generally offer reassurance.

Membership is renewed by a $20 subscription in July each year.

A list of other support groups throughout Australia is listed after Chapter 13.

6
THE NOT-SO-MERRY-GO-ROUND

By the time you get to a treatment cycle, you would have been through preliminary routine investigations including blood tests, semen analysis and counselling.

The blood tests you and your partner should have had include Rubella—all female patients are tested for Rubella (German Measles) immunity. If there is no natural immunity, you must have a vaccination before starting treatment to avoid the risk of rubella damaging the foetus.

You are also tested for Hepatitis B as carriers must be detected to protect other patients and staff.

We would have tested your hormone levels—prolactin and Follicle Stimulating Hormone levels are tested around Day 8 of your cycle to ensure that these are normal.

Female sperm antibodies are checked in the blood. This is necessary as blood from the wife maybe added to the fluid the eggs are grown in, to assist embryo development. Occasionally, the blood contains antibodies to the husband's sperm which will prevent fertilisation. If the blood is sperm antibody positive, it is discarded and a donor's blood is used.

HIV is now the internationally accepted way of classifying the AIDS virus and stands for Human Immunodeficiency Virus. We do this test because pregnancy increases the death rate dramatically to a female who is infected with the virus. The second reason is the risk to the medical staff who handle body fluids from a large population on a daily basis. Naturally, we would need to take special precautions with samples from HIV positive patients.

Like HIV, samples from patients with hepatitis are hazardous to staff unless special precautions are taken. It is more infectious than HIV, although the death rate is much lower. Both husband and wife are tested. Victorian legislation requires that all potential IVF couples attend a counselling session prior to starting treatment. At present, this is only available to couples on an individual basis although we do cater for small groups of up to four couples.

When you have been accepted on to the program, you may need to wait for up to four months before treatment begins.

You can make use of this waiting time by making sure all preliminary investigations are completed and do your best to get fit and healthy. Eat a healthy, well balanced diet with adequate protein, carbohydrate and fibre.

Stop smoking and reduce your alcohol intake. We recommend that you stop drinking alcohol prior to pregnancy. Smoking increases the risk of miscarriage and alcohol may harm the foetus.

Being overweight can reduce your chance of success, so if you need to lose weight, use this waiting time to do it.

It is important that you inform the clinic of any change of address or telephone number as this avoids any disappointment if we are unable to contact you. We also ask that if you decide not to go ahead with the treatment, let us know so that other couples can be treated instead.

Likewise, if you conceive while on the waiting list, please let us know. If you miscarry or have an ectopic pregnancy, this will not prejudice your place on the waiting list.

If you are taking medications, make sure you ask if these will be necessary during your treatment cycle. We appreciate that many drugs need to be continued, but it may be best to postpone your IVF treatment while taking short-term medication. Do not stop medication without specific advice from your clinician. This also applies to male partners as some medications are known to reduce sperm counts.

In Vitro Fertilisation (IVF)

Having been through all of that, you are now ready to start your treatment cycle. What does it involve? There are six basic steps in an IVF treatment cycle:

- Follicle growth (stimulated cycle using drugs)
- Ovulation timing (based on blood tests and ultrasound scan)
- Collecting the eggs from the follicles (this is the egg pick-up)
- Fertilisation of the eggs with the husband's sperm
- Embryo transfer to the uterus (ET)
- Pregnancy test (a blood test carried out on day 28).

Follicle Growth and Ovulation Timing

Follicle growth and ovulation timing depend upon the development of a satisfactory hormone protocol to stimulate the ovaries. Ovulation is triggered by the injection of a hormone, HCG (Human Chorionic Gonadotrophin).

BOOST or FLARE protocol

(Buserelin Oocyte Stimulation Regimen)

Buserelin or Lupron (Leuprolide Acetate) which act in the same way, are similar to gonadotrophin releasing hormone. The term 'flare' is also used to describe this method as the drug causes an initial flare of ovarian action. The drugs then prevent natural ovulation so fewer blood tests are needed and eggs are not lost by ovulation before egg pick up.

This new protocol was introduced to maximise the pregnancy rate potential for couples coming through IVF and GIFT treatments.

Some of the ancillary benefits to patients include:
- simplifying a previously technically involved treatment cycle;
- preventing the natural LH surge which occurs with the onset of ovulation. This normally results in patients being cancelled from continuing a treatment cycle as ovulation has already taken place;
- lowering the number of visits, blood collections and waiting time for patients.

Pre-treatment investigation and consultation

Two weeks before the first day of her period, the woman rings the clinic to make an appointment to see a clinician.

The woman and her husband meet the clinician during the week before her period is due and at this consultation the patient is given a summary of her proposed treatment cycle. As well, a baseline vaginal ultrasound is taken (to check for cysts, endometrioma, polyps or fibroids).

Treatment

Day 1	The woman rings IMC to advise first day of period.
Day 2	She begins injections of Lupron once a day in the evening and continues this through to Day 12 approximately, or to the day of the HCG injection which triggers ovulation.
Day 3	She begins intramuscular Metrodin (FSH) or HMG (Human Menopausal Gonadotrophin, which is both FSH and LH) daily from Day 3 until Day 12 approximately, or until the day of the HCG injection.
Day 8	The woman comes to IMC for an interview with the clinician. A blood test is taken and the woman undergoes a vaginal ultrasound (to check for follicular development). If follicle measurement and hormone levels are good, the HCG injection may be booked now. If follicular size is poor/small, the Metrodin or HMG dose may be increased.

At this stage it is possible for a patient to be cancelled from continuing the treatment cycle. If so, the woman is contacted by a clinician and the appropriate reason for cancellation is given over the telephone. The woman and her husband are invited to the clinic for a consultation with the clinician the next day, should they desire this.

For patients continuing with the treatment cycle:

Day 10	Again the woman sees the clinician, has a blood test and another vaginal ultrasound. The HCG injection can

	be booked from Day 10 and the oocyte collection is arranged for a time 36 hours after this injection.
Day 13	The rest of the procedure takes place as in a routine IVF procedure i.e. egg culture, fertilisation and transfer.
Day 14–28	Injections of HCG or vaginal progesterone pessaries may be required to ensure the best conditions for implantation of the embryo.
Day 28	(Or Day 14 post retrieval). A blood test for pregnancy is taken—E2, P4 and HCG are measured.

Costs associated with BOOST:

All costs associated with IVF changed from November 1990 as new Medicare numbers are being introduced. The out-of-pocket costs currently being paid by patients are about $300.

Down Regulation Protocol

The patient has Lupron or Buserelin (GnRH-like drugs) for 2–3 weeks to stop ovarian function before stimulating the ovary with gonadotrophins, HMG or FSH (metrodin).

Down regulation is preferred when BOOST or FLARE are ineffective, or cysts form with stimulation.

Clomid Protocol

Only chlomiphene is used. One or two eggs develop, the success rate is lower, 8 per cent, but only one blood test and ultrasound is done.

Natural Cycle

No drugs are used and only one blood test and ultrasound is required. Success rate is 4 per cent per treatment.

Egg pick-up

The egg pick-up is by vaginal ultrasound or laparoscopy.

For the pick-up to succeed, three things are required—accurate timing so that the eggs are sufficiently mature, accessibility of the ovaries to the vaginal needle or laparoscope and a good egg collection technique.

Nearly all women have egg pick-up by vaginal ultrasound. A light anaesthesia, called neurolept, or local anaesthesia is used. A small minority of women require no anaesthesia.

A probe contained in an ultrasound transmitter is passed into the vagina, and a picture of the ovary is seen on a TV screen.

A fine needle is passed from the vagina into the follicles to collect eggs, the needle being directed by matching its movement on the television screen.

Mature eggs are mostly in follicles over the size of 15mm. Only follicles over 12mm are aspirated.

By means of a vacuum pressure device which the surgeon operates by foot, the fluid is sucked from the follicle through the needle, and placed in a flat glass dish. The amount of fluid is usually about one to 15 millilitres and is the colour of straw. The egg itself within the fluid is only one-tenth of a mm in size and is invisible to the naked eye. However, as it is usually surrounded by mucous and a layer of cells about one mm in diameter, the whole complex may be seen as a tiny white speck in the fluid.

This fluid is taken to the laboratory and a scientist or a specially-trained laboratory technician immediately examines it under high magnification.

Sometimes the egg is not collected because it is attached to the wall of the follicle and is not in the free fluid which has been removed. When the technician reports that no egg is present in the fluid collected, the surgeon may inject fluid into the follicle until it reaches its original size. The fluid is then sucked out in the hope that any egg that has adhered to the wall of the follicle will become detached.

Eggs collected by this technique of flushing the follicle are less likely to be fully mature as one of the natural changes that occurs prior to ovulation is that the egg becomes free-floating in the fluid of the follicle. Nevertheless, pregnancies have followed follicle flushing. If an egg cannot be found after several flushings, the search is abandoned.

Sometimes ovulation has already occurred. This is recognized by the fact that the follicle or follicles previously identified using ultrasound have burst.

But all is not lost. The egg may drop from the ovary into the pouch behind the uterus, and can sometimes be collected. Two things are done. The ruptured follicle is flushed, as the egg may still be stuck within it, and the fluid from the pouch behind the uterus is sucked out and examined.

Eggs are successfully collected from about 60–70 per cent of follicles, but sometimes no eggs are collected or each follicle yields an egg.

Very rarely egg collection fails by this method and laparoscopy is required.

Women having an egg pick-up by laparoscopy are given a general anaesthetic. As pregnancies have occurred following relatively prolonged general anaesthesia, it is not thought that the anaesthetic affects the eggs.

Normally when a laparoscopy is performed solely to examine the ovaries, two incisions are made in the abdomen. A cut, a few millimetres long, is made in the umbilicus (belly button) and a telescope-like instrument with its own light attached—the laparoscope—is introduced so that the ovaries can be viewed. The second puncture site is usually made in the lower abdomen along the hair-line and a fine forcep is passed through. This allows the pelvic organs to be manipulated and positioned appropriately.

When carrying out a laparoscopy for the purpose of picking up eggs, a third puncture site is made between the first and second incisions. This enables the surgeon to pass a teflon-coated needle into each mature follicle and to remove the fluid and the egg it contains.

By looking through the laparoscope held in one hand, and manipulating each ovary into various positions with the other, the surgeon can identify any ripe follicles. These look like button mushrooms and are 1.5 to 2.5 cm in size. They usually have a thin wall, through which the fluid is visible.

The needle is passed through the wall of the follicle as slowly and carefully as possible in order to prevent fluid leakage or damage to the egg. Eggs are collected as for the ultrasound method.

Advances in the technique of egg collection and the increasing skill of the surgeons, has resulted in a situation where, in nearly all patients, at least one egg is collected. The average number collected is seven eggs.

The next step is to separate the egg from the fluid that surrounds it. If the fluid is clear, this is not difficult. But if blood is present, and particularly if a clot is formed around the egg and its surrounding cells, separating one from the other is not easy. Fortunately, the egg has some elasticity and will withstand minor distortion. But any strong manipulation may lead to damage.

Egg culture

Once the egg is free, it is quickly placed in the culture fluid, which is then placed in an incubator. This provides suitable conditions for sustaining the health of the egg; temperature and humidity are controlled precisely and a clean environment is assured over the surface of the culture fluid.

For the next two to 12 hours, the egg is left undisturbed in the hope that it will mature, as it would before natural ovulation. All eggs are used for IVF.

If an excess of eggs are collected, a woman may consider donating one or more eggs to another woman who cannot produce eggs. Then IVF is carried out using sperm cells from the recipient's husband.

In order for sperm cells to be capable of penetrating the egg, they have to undergo a change from the state they are in at the time of ejaculation. This change, called capacitation, normally occurs as the sperm cells pass through the genital tract, and involves the shedding of the outer coat of the sperm head.

Capacitation has a number of other benefits. It results in increased sperm cell activity and they therefore move more vigorously. Also, the chemicals released during capacitation may assist in sperm cell penetration of the layer of cells and the coat surrounding the egg.

In the human, inducing capacitation is quite simple, in contrast to the situation in many other species. It is achieved by washing the sperm cells twice in a simple solution and leaving them in culture fluid for one to two hours. Then the sperm cells are examined under a microscope to ensure that they are still active and those required for fertilisation are collected. This involves a relatively simple selection procedure as the most healthy and active sperm cells tend to be concentrated in the upper part of the culture fluid. For men with poor sperm counts or motility, special methods are used to collect the best sperm from the sample.

Fertilisation

Fertilisation and sperm growth occur in fluid similar to, but simpler than, human plasma. Attempts to improve the media are continuing by adding cells from the lining of tubes which may assist fertilisation and embryo development or by adding special growth promoting factors. About 50,000 sperm cells are placed with the egg, in the procedure known as insemination. More sperm are used if the sperm are defective or antibodies are present.

The egg and the sperm cells are then returned to the incubator, in the expectation that a single sperm cell will penetrate the egg. This is the first of a series of steps in the process of fertilisation.

The sperm cell passes through the outer layer of cells and mucous surrounding the egg, and then through the coat and substance of the egg. This normally takes several hours and requires both the action of chemical substances from the sperm cell, together with its own physical thrust from movement of the tail.

As soon as one sperm cell has passed into the core of the egg, a barrier to further sperm cell entry is usually created by chemicals released by the egg. If more than one sperm cell enters, fertilisation may be abnormal or unsuccessful, or embryo development may proceed abnormally.

This is one disadvantage of the IVF procedure as—since a larger number of sperm cells are in a position to enter the egg than in the orthodox situation—it would seem more likely that several sperm cells could enter simultaneously, before the barrier to further sperm cell entry becomes effective. This occurs in about 3 per cent of embryos resulting from IVF and these are discarded as they may result in abnormal development.

The result of penetration by the sperm cell is that its genetic material combines with the genetic material of the egg, thus providing the blueprint that is essential for the development of a new human life. This occurs at about 22 hours and is called syngamy. When fertilisation is delayed beyond 28 hours the risk of chromosomal abnormalities are high, 80 per cent, so these embryos are discarded. We have permission to biopsy embryos. This will distinguish the normal from abnormal embryos without harming the embryo thus saving the 20 per cent of normal embryos occurring after delayed fertilisation.

With the GIFT procedure, fertilisation occurs in the fallopian tube as it would in an unassisted conception. The eggs and sperm are not brought into contact with each other until they are in the fallopian tube, so no human interference with actual conception has occurred. Thus GIFT can overcome some of the objections to the IVF procedure—it does not "create life in the laboratory". It does not intervene in fertilisation. Of course, intervention in procreation has occurred, but in a more limited way.

As with IVF, couples who have GIFT may have additional injections of HCG so that hours after the operation is over, the couple are free to go home, to wait.

Embryo growth and assessment

The embryo so formed moves through a series of cell divisions, and about 48 hours after insemination it has grown from one cell to eight.

The quality of health of the embryo is judged by the speed at which it develops as well as on its appearance. In a normal embryo, the cells are regular in outline and approximately equal in size. Irregularity of cells or distortion of shape indicates abnormality. Fragments may appear in the ovary which indicate reduced viability. Experience shows that an embryo with an abnormal appearance or very slow growth no longer has the potential to form human life. Since it no longer has this potential, it is certified as dead and, as in the case of adult material in which death has occurred with no apparent cause, an examination may be carried out to try to determine the reason.

The information gained is not always conclusive, but sometimes it is possible to determine the cause of an abnormal embryo.

Early in the history of the Melbourne program, embryo transfers were carried out at the eight or sixteen cell stage of development. It is now clear that the uterus will accept embryos consisting of one, two or four cells, and pregnancies have followed at these early stages. This early transfer has some advantages; it avoids a prolonged period in the culture fluid, which may adversely affect the embryo, and once the transfer is made, the possibility of environmental contamination of the embryo culture fluid is removed.

In the Monash/Epworth program, the human embryo is transferred at the two or four-cell stage but other IVF groups are as successful transferring more mature embryos at the eight to sixteen-cell stage. If fertilisation does not occur, the egg is studied to find out why and, whenever possible, an explanation is offered to the couple concerned. Sometimes a cause is evident, and steps to overcome the problem may be taken during the next treatment attempt. The most common cause is poor egg or sperm quality.

The best chance of becoming pregnant is achieved if four or more mature eggs are removed from the ovaries and several embryos develop.

The policy of fertilising all mature eggs sometimes results in formation of four or more embryos. In this situation, both the couple and the treatment team face an ethical dilemma.

The couple may wish to have two or three embryos transferred, but not for example, four or five, because of the very small chance of quadruplets or quintuplets. In general, couples are advised to accept two or three embryos.

Four or more embryos are only transferred if one or two embryos are not classified as good quality or the patient is over 40 years.

The chance of pregnancy increases from 7 per cent for one, 14 per cent for two and 23 per cent for three embryos transferred. The likelihood of twins when two embryos are transferred is 15 per cent. When three embryos are transferred the chance of pregnancy is 23 per cent, and the chance of multiple pregnancy about 20 per cent, including the possibility of triplets.

Although twins are associated with slightly increased risks, such as premature labour and a higher mortality rate, the prospect of two babies rather than one is attractive to most couples. Having been infertile for some years, they appreciate that this may be their only chance of establishing a family.

The risk of triplets can be avoided by only transferring two good quality embryos.

Freezing embryos

The dilemma remains about what to do with excess embryos. In nearly all IVF programs, embryos are frozen in liquid nitrogen for use by the couple at a later date.

Freezing of embryos was established in 1984 and, by the end of 1988, 52 babies had been born in Melbourne as a result of this technical breakthrough.

Many more embryos are now frozen as there has been an increase in the number of eggs collected—the average is six—and the embryo freezing procedure has gradually improved.

The stored embryos can be thawed and transferred in a subsequent menstrual cycle if the initial transfer of fresh embryos fails. Or, if the first transfer attempt results in a continuing pregnancy, the embryos can be thawed a year or two later in a bid to achieve a second pregnancy.

Embryos can also be frozen and stored if the initial transfer cannot be carried out because of sudden illness, bleeding from the uterus, or if transfer through the cervix proves too difficult.

One way to avoid the formation of excess embryos is to limit the number of eggs collected or used in fertilisation attempts to the exact number required for transfer.

This has several disadvantages, however. The best eggs may be left in the ovary or, even if collected, they may not be selected for fertilisation. Also, ripe egg follicles remaining in the ovary may develop into painful cysts.

To provide patients in our program with the greatest possible chance of pregnancy, all the eggs collected are fertilised, and the number of embryos requested by the patient transferred immediately. Any embryos not transferred at this time are preserved for the couple by freezing until they can be used.

If the eggs capable of forming a baby could be identified by microscopic examination and/or other tests, freezing may not be necessary. But in the absence of this capability, we regard attempted freezing as an ethical obligation. Even when the woman is pregnant after the initial treatment, she can attempt further pregnancy with the frozen embryos left over.

The freeze-thaw procedure involves the use of a chemical to help preserve embryos during the freezing process, which takes several hours. Only about 60-70 per cent of embryos survive the freeze-thaw process.

When more than half the cells survive, the embryo is transferred. The evidence available indicates that even one cell of an early embryo may be capable of forming a normal baby.

Researchers are attempting to improve the success rate of freeze-thawing as only about 9 per cent of thawed embryos that are transferred result in pregnancy. Most patients have two frozen-thawed embryos transferred at one time, the pregnancy rate being 18 per cent per transfer.

The use of a chemical preservant and the physical effect on the embryo of the freeze-thaw process itself have raised questions about whether developmental abnormalities are likely to result. Studies of embryos and babies produced after freeze-thawing indicate that there is no increased risk of abnormalities. In sheep and cattle, similar freeze-thaw techniques do not lead to abnormal offspring.

Patients having embryos frozen sign a consent form stating they understand the risks of the procedure. In addition, the couples indicate their wishes for their stored embryos should they die, become ill, divorce or change their mind about having another attempt at pregnancy. The majority of those who do not wish to attempt another pregnancy opt to donate their embryos to be used for research or be destroyed.

One advantage of freezing is that the system of transferring frozen embryos in a natural cycle is more simple than a full treatment cycle which involves stimulation. The natural cycle is less strenuous, physically, with no injection and few blood tests.

There are two ways of running a frozen embryo transfer cycle. One is for the patient to have blood or urine tests to determine when ovulation is occurring. Urine kits can be used by the patient at home avoiding hospital visits. Embryos are then put back the number of days after ovulation to coincide with the age of the embryo. For example, if the embryo is three days old, the transfer would be three days after ovulation takes place in the natural cycle.

The second way avoids the need for blood or urine tests. The patient takes oestrogen tablets to supress ovulation before embryo transfer. Progesterone is given after the embryo is put back. The disadvantage of this method is that the patient needs to continue with progesterone after the pregnancy is established, for approximately 4 to 6 weeks. It is more expensive because of the cost of the drugs, and less popular.

One in four patients have frozen embryos transferred. The chance of pregnancy from the original stimulated cycle is about doubled.

Many patients ask me how soon after a failed IVF attempt can they undergo a frozen embryo transfer. This is your choice but we do suggest you need at least one month to recover physically and emotionally.

A rest is sometimes necessary hormonally because after a stimulation cycle, you may not ovulate the following cycle.

Freezing of embryos has opened up a whole range of problems and possibilities. As yet we don't know how long an embryo can survive in a frozen state, and it is not unlikely that one day a mother could pass on her frozen embryos to an infertile daughter. Frozen embryos have been used successfully in other species 10–15 years later.

There is no limit on the number of embryos each patient may have frozen but we always recommend that a patient have the frozen embryos transferred before going on to another treatment cycle.

The only exception would be if the frozen embryo was not of good quality and then we would suggest delaying transfer to see if a better embryo can be obtained from another treatment cycle. Subsequently, two embryos would be transferred in one cycle.

Freezing of eggs is more difficult and only two pregnancies resulting from the use of thawed eggs had occurred to the end of 1986. Because the chromosomes of the mature egg are more unstable than those of the embryo, it is possible that chromosomal damage could occur more readily due to the effects of the chemical preservants and/or the freezing process.

In mice, freeze-thawing of eggs has resulted in more abnormal embryos than expected. The technique of freeze-thawing of eggs thus requires improvement in human embryos before it can be considered safe. Legislative limitation of embryo studies has stymied efforts to ensure the safety of the technique involved.

Yet freezing of eggs has great potential as there are fewer ethical problems involved in the freezing of excess eggs than of excess embryos. Refinement of the technique and validation of its safety would also enable the storage of eggs for subsequent donation to women with no eggs due to absent or damaged ovaries, or to women with unsatisfactory eggs carrying a risk of genetic disease. The eggs of women with early stage pelvic diseases such as endometriosis, cysts or infections, could also be stored as an insurance against the subsequent loss of both ovaries. Eggs might even be stored by young women wishing to defer childbearing to a later date when changes in their eggs might increase the risk of Down's Syndrome in a child.

The embryo transfer

Although the transfer of the embryo to the uterus is a critical procedure, the technique is reasonably simple.

One to three days after the sperm cells are placed with the egg, the scientist decides whether the embryo is normal in appearance and growing well enough for a transfer to take place.

The transfer usually takes places 30 to 48 hours after the sperm cells are added to the egg, by which stage the embryo comprises 2 to 4 cells.

An hour before the proposed time of the transfer the patient is offered a tranquillizer. Although it is a pity to dampen feelings at this time, some patients are over anxious and find it difficult to relax sufficiently to enable a smooth, gentle transfer. It is also possible that anxiety may make the uterus more active by stimulating the release of certain hormones, and this may increase the risk of embryo expulsion.

At one time patients were given a drug to block uterine activity in the hope that this would improve the success of embryo transfer, but this was not obviously effective so the practice has been abandoned.

The embryo transfer takes place in the operating theatre, as the Victorian Law states that these procedures must be done in a hospital. It would be equally safe and more pleasant for couples if the procedure was done in an informal, more congenial atmosphere rather than in an operating theatre.

In a room close to the operating theatre, the embryo is placed in a tiny drop of fluid which is transferred to a fine tube about 1mm in diameter. Although placement of the embryo in this drop of fluid requires considerable skill, it is extremely rare that an embryo is damaged during the procedure: the scientists practise the technique on mouse embryos until they are expert enough to handle human embryos.

It is important that subsequent events occur as quickly and gently as possible. An embryo in such a tiny drop of fluid may be affected adversely by cold air or evaporation of the fluid which surrounds it, and this could lead to critical changes in its chemistry.

While the embryo is made ready the patient lies on her back with her legs in stirrups, or supports, and covered by drapes. The doctor inserts a speculum—the metal instrument shaped to fit the vagina—and exposes the cervix. The position and size of the uterus is checked in order to determine the best method for passing the tube containing the embryo into it. Any excess fluid on the cervix is removed because, if this is introduced into the cervix as the catheter is passed, it may stick to the embryo and prevent it implanting in the uterus.

When all is ready, the embryo is brought into the operating theatre. Working together, the doctor and scientist pass the tube or catheter through the vagina and then through the cervix a short distance into the uterus.

The best position for releasing the embryo is not known for certain, but it seems reasonable that this should occur at about the place where the fallopian tube meets the uterus, which is a half to one centimetre from the top of the uterus.

This position is accurately determined from a measurement of the length of the uterus made during an ultrasound scan earlier in the cycle. By marking the distance on the catheter and subtracting a centimetre, the embryo is assured of reasonable placement.

Before the embryos are injected into the uterus, the position of the catheter in the uterus may be checked by ultrasound.

The catheter is passed slowly and gently, as any forceful manipulation against the wall of the uterus may cause bleeding or stimulate uterine activity. Either of these may thwart the transfer attempt.

If the catheter sticks as it passes through the cervix, it is manipulated in various directions in a bid to find a clear passage.

The technique of embryo transfer requires practice and experience as the natural tendency is to complete the procedure as quickly as possible in order to protect the embryo.

Often, the catheter is passed inside a guiding sheath which helps to direct it through the cervix and uterus. In recent years also, improvements to catheters have resulted in easier transfers. A surgeon may choose from a range of catheters, since one may be more suitable than others in a particular situation.

Women who have had a vaginal delivery previously are at an advantage here. For childbirth dilates the cervix to some extent and the catheter thus passes more easily into the uterus.

A trial transfer is sometimes carried out before the treatment cycle. This has several advantages: the patient is acquainted with the procedure and is often more confident and less anxious about it, and if difficulties arise during the trial transfer, the cause of the problem may be identified and preventative measures may be possible at the time of the actual transfer. For example, anxious patients in whom the vagina contracts during examination, can be given an epidural anaesthetic. Or if the catheter will not pass easily through the cervix, the patient can have a dilatation of the cervix in the treatment cycle. This involves a day in hospital and a local or general anaesthetic and results in an easier transfer.

Sometimes the transfer is impossible or doomed to failure. For example, if bleeding occurs in the uterus, it may form a clot around the embryo preventing implantation; or else the embryo may be washed through the cervix with the blood.

Rarely it is impossible to pass the catheter through the cervix. In this circumstance, there are several alternatives: either the embryo is replaced in the culture fluid and a further attempt is made the next day, or it is frozen for transfer at a later date.

The catheter is withdrawn slowly in order to minimise the chance of the embryo moving along an artificial track left by it.

One obvious disadvantage of transferring the embryo through the cervix is that the catheter disrupts the plug of mucous that would tend normally to assist in the retention of the embryo.

After the transfer procedure, the catheter is inspected in the laboratory under the microscope to ensure that the embryo has indeed been delivered into the patient.

Ultrasound guidance during transfer may assist or improve the technique and is used in most patients.

Care and assessment after transfer

Patients walk in and out of the embryo transfer room as it is thought that the embryo rapidly takes position in the adhesive type of secretion lining the uterus.

In the conventional situation no special care is taken, and embryos are thought to implant after three days in the uterus.

Patients may experience bloating from distension of the bowel, abdominal pain from ovarian bruising or blood in the pelvis, or tiredness. These symptoms may require rest or use of mild analgesics.

Couples can have sexual intercourse after transfer. Tests on the 12th and 14th days after transfer will indicate whether the pregnancy is likely to continue. Once a pregnancy is verified, weekly hormone tests follow.

Low levels of pregnancy hormones are associated with an increased risk of natural abortion, or ectopic pregnancy, and couples are warned of this possibility. Both in the conventional system and the test-tube procedure, abortions occur most often before or around the time of the next period. Women are usually unaware of such abortions.

Once the pregnancy has continued for eight weeks following IVF and Embryo Transfer, the chances of a miscarriage occurring are very similar to that of the conventional situation.

GIFT procedure (Gametes In Fallopian Tube)

Gametes (sperm and egg) are collected and placed immediately into the fallopian tubes.

The GIFT procedure is for women who do not have tubal damage or disease, and unfortunately tubal involvement is thought to be responsible for infertility in up to 30 per cent of infertile women.

GIFT offers a better chance, if your infertility is not due to problems with the fallopian tubes, but it still involves anxiety, stress and emotional drain on the couple involved in the program.

It may be suitable for couples with male infertility, success rates often being better than with IVF.

The collection of eggs for GIFT is carried out by vaginal ultrasound under light anaesthesia. All large follicles are aspirated. Usually a maximum of two to four eggs are used in the procedure. If a woman is over 40 years or the husband's sperm is abnormal up to six eggs may be transferred. If more than the required number of eggs are collected, the couple decide beforehand how they are to be dealt with.

Excess eggs can be used for IVF and the embryos frozen which can be used in a subsequent cycle if pregnancy does not occur.

Eggs can be discarded, or in some programs they can be donated to another couple for use in either GIFT or IVF.

If the new technique of ovum freezing becomes available, it will offer the chance to freeze excess eggs which could then be used for a future GIFT procedure in which ovarian stimulation had not occurred, or could be used for an IVF with the embryo transfer in an unstimulated cycle.

One significant difference between GIFT and IVF is that for GIFT the sperm is collected before the eggs. With IVF, the husband is not asked to provide sperm until a few hours after the eggs have been collected because it has been found that fertilisation occurs more readily if the eggs have been left for a few hours to mature. But GIFT needs to have the sperm ready when the eggs are available, so sperm is collected at least one hour prior to the operation. This can be advantageous if the man has found it difficult to collect sperm by masturbation in that his wife can be available to help.

It is possible to allow the couple to have intercourse prior to the operation and catch the sperm in a special condom (ordinary condoms are spermicidal). This might overcome the objection some couples have to IVF because of religious beliefs opposed to masturbation. However, the pressure to perform might be so intense that intercourse and ejaculation could be difficult—if it's hard to time your love life by the thermometer, think of the pressure with a fully equipped and staffed operating theatre waiting for you!

Assume, however, that the ideal procedure is underway; several eggs have been collected, and a sample of the husband's sperm is available. As soon as the eggs are identified by the scientist in the operating theatre or adjacent laboratory, three eggs are drawn up into a very fine teflon-lined catheter, followed by about 50-100,000 sperm which have been washed and centrifuged to collect the best sperm and allowed to mature for about two hours for capacitation to occur.

The surgeon then threads the fine catheter into the fallopian tube and deposits the eggs and the sperm. If both fallopian tubes are accessable and patent, and if there are enough eggs, the same procedure is repeated on the other side. The GIFT has been made—gamete intrafallopian transfer has occurred, the incisions are closed and the woman is transferred from the operating theatre to the recovery room and then to her own bed. The woman usually goes home the same day, unless pain or vomiting prevents this.

GIFT can now be done by collecting the eggs with vaginal ultrasound, and then passing a catheter with eggs and sperm inside, from the vagina through the cavity of the uterus to the tubes, and depositing the sperm and eggs there. This does not require laparoscopy or general anaesthetic. The success rate is not yet as high as the laparoscopy GIFT procedure.

In Australia, the success rate per GIFT procedure is between 25 per cent and 40 per cent. Not all patients beginning the program will proceed to laparoscopy—only about 80 per cent will have eggs collected, and less than half of those who have eggs and sperm deposited in the fallopian tubes will find they do get pregnant.

But the maze is a shorter one—waiting to see if the eggs fertilise and the embryos develop properly is no longer a process that can be observed, and the possibility of difficulty in replacing the embryos has been avoided. Whether fertilisation has occurred and implantation has taken place is not known until the period is due. The chances of achieving a pregnancy is much higher than with IVF, possibly because the fallopian tube provides the best possible environment for fertilisation and development of the embryo.

Further treatments

If a pregnancy does not occur after the IVF or GIFT procedure, it is important for couples to see their doctor so that the situation can be discussed and a decision made about a further treatment attempt.

In the Monash/Epworth program, couples usually have three or four treatment attempts although some have continued and become pregnant after ten to twelve treatments. The success rate is similar up to the fifth attempt.

The time interval between treatments is best decided by couples after discussion with their doctor. Some couples prefer to have the attempts within a short period of time so that the matter can be dealt with as quickly as possible. They can then organise their lives according to whether a pregnancy has, or has not, occurred. Couples are advised however, to allow one clear month between each attempt.

Others prefer to space the attempts at yearly intervals either to recuperate from each attempt, to save money for the next attempt, or to improve their chances of success—assuming that the success rate for the procedure will improve each year.

Deciding when to abandon treatment is a difficult decision, especially after a lengthy period of treatment in which high hopes are invested. In making the decision, partners should be clear about the treatments that have been attempted and whether any other treatment has a reasonable chance of success.

During the treatment, partners may become overwrought and sometimes it is a good idea to defer the treatment until the emotional and physical energy is restored.

When all possible treatments have been offered and failed, it is important that couples understand why this is so, and to face the actuality of not being able to have children of their own.

Treatment check list

- Record the first day of each menstrual period in your diary while on the waiting list.
- Leave an address and phone number for contact of both partners during the treatment cycle.
- Avoid jellies or creams for masturbation during collection of semen samples, as these may kill sperm cells.
- Make sure you understand the instructions concerning injection doses outside the clinic.
- Avoid excess exercise soon after the treatment procedure.
- Rest if you become very tired or have abdominal pain.
- Contact the clinic if you have any questions about your health, including a fever, use of drugs or pain.

7
TAKING DRUGS

I understand that many of you would be concerned over adverse reports about the use of fertility drugs.

There is no scientific evidence supporting claims that the drugs may cause cancer, premature menopause or ageing.

To discuss why we use fertility drugs on the IVF program, it is necessary to start at the beginning. Obviously the main aim of the fertility drug is to encourage more than one egg to ripen. This is done for two reasons: to increase your chances of producing at least one healthy embryo for transfer and hopefully a desired pregnancy. The second is that we need to know when a patient is going to require egg pick-up so that the operating theatre can be booked in advance. We need to be aware of this so theatre staff and other hospital requirements can be catered for.

On our program we use three methods to stimulate the ovaries: Lupron or Buserelin with HMG or Metrodin (BOOST) or down-regulation using Lupron followed by HMG or Metrodin: Clomid with HMG or Metrodin.

The first two mentioned were the most commonly used and the use of Clomid with HMG is being phased out because of the better results we are achieving with the combination of Lupron and HMG or Metrodin.

We have carried out a number of clinical trials establishing the effectiveness of Lupron and HMG. It is a popular choice of drug because it requires only one or two blood tests over the whole treatment, rather than the twice daily bloods required for patients on Clomid.

Lupron downregulation is being used in patients who do not respond to the BOOST or FLARE regime because we find it is more effective in stimulating ovulation in these patients.

Lupron is given as a daily injection. This drug must be kept refrigerated—making life a little difficult for those patients still working—and like Clomid, starts on day one to two of your cycle.

The HMG injections begin the day after you start either Buserelin, Lupron or Clomid.

We know that Lupron, Buserelin and Clomid have side effects. For Buserelin these include hot flushes, tiredness and at times, headaches. Clomid also causes hot flushes, headaches and nausea and occasionally blurred vision. You may be unfortunate enough to suffer all symptoms or, like some patients, lucky enough not to even notice you are taking the drug.

The important rule is not to be frightened to contact your doctor or a member of the team should any side effects cause you alarm. It may simply be that the dosage is too high for you.

HMG contains both Follicle Stimulating Hormone (FSH) and Luteinizing Hormone (LH) and the injections are used to stimulate the ovaries with the aim of producing more than one egg. These usually start the day after Clomid or Lupron/Buserelin and are given for five or more days.

Metrodin contains mostly Follicle Stimulating Hormone (FSH). Like other injections used during the cycle, we are encouraging husbands, friends or even patients to administer these injections themselves.

This will obviate the need for extra trips to the hospital—which we appreciate are time-consuming and annoying—and soon blood tests will be taken at "satellite centres" situated around the state to help both country and city patients eliminate the need to spend time travelling and waiting to have blood taken. Our long-term plan would be to use these satellite centres to do everything but the actual egg pick-up so that the patients require only one visit to hospital during each cycle.

Patients with hormone disorders may require the use of different drugs. We determine this by asking each patient to undergo several hormone estimations prior to starting treatment to detect any abnormalities.

When an imbalance of FSH and LH production occurs, Lupron or Buserelin may be used to stop natural FSH and LH production and the ovary is then stimulated by injections of Metrodin which stimulates the release of FSH more than Luteinizing Hormone (LH) from the pituitary gland.

Blocking ovarian function by the use of Lupron or Buserelin, which is a chemical similar to gonadotrophin releasing hormone, before giving pituitary hormones to stimulate the ovary is the preferred treatment for patients who do not respond to the simultaneous regimes of Clomid-HMG or Buserelin-HMG. This is known as downregulation and about 15 per cent of our patients end up using this method. The Lupron is used for 2-3 weeks before the ovary is down regulated (stops functioning) when HMG or Metrodin (FSH) is commenced.

The greatest possible care is taken in determining the appropriate dosage of fertility drugs. If the ovaries are over-stimulated, cysts may form in the ovaries which are very painful and can cause bleeding.

If you have any concerns at all while taking a fertility drug, alert a team member.

Strictly-controlled monitoring is also important in preventing an over-stimulation of the ovaries.

If overstimulation occurs the ovaries swell, cause pain from cyst formation, and fluid accumulates in the abdomen. This problem may require rest, occasionally admission to hospital and one to three weeks to recover. Pregnancy is more likely in women suffering overstimulation.

The blood tests are one of the most disliked functions in the program. Why do we need them? It is necessary to know accurately when ovulation will occur so that the ripe eggs can be picked up just before they are released from the ovaries. Each treatment involves two or four blood tests.

We need to monitor the progress of the maturing egg and this is done by ultrasound, oestrogen, progesterone and LH hormone measurements.

Previous menstrual cycle lengths are taken into account and the information about the rate of the egg ripening determines when an injection of another fertility drug, Human Choroinic Gonadotrophin (HCG) is given to complete the ripening of the eggs. This is given 36 hours before egg pick up.

Here is a brief summary of the drugs used, their side effects and what they contain:

Clomiphene Citrate (Clomid):

Taken orally, these tablets act on the hypothalamus, pituitary and ovary to initiate ovulation. The pituitary gland produces hormones stimulating the ovary and Clomid also has a direct and favourable effect on the ovary.

Because Clomid helps the body to function naturally, over-stimulation, resulting in multiple birth, is less likely.

Side effects: Hot flushes, abdominal discomfort or bloating, blurred vision (rare), nausea, nervous tension, depression, fatigue, dizziness and light-headedness, insomnia, headache and breast soreness. The drug should be stopped if blurred vision occurs.

Buserelin/Lupron:

These are chemicals similar to gonadotrophin releasing hormone, taken via a nasal spray four times a day or by injection. They allow us to better pick the time of egg pick-up because it prevents premature ovulation.

Buserelin and Lupron have two actions, to 'boost' pituitary stimulation of the ovaries on the first 2–3 days of use and block pituitary ovarian functions with more prolonged use.

In this way these drugs increase hormone levels for 2–3 days and after that, stop pituitary hormone release and the release of the egg.

The dual action is important in the BOOST technique.

We also use Buserelin or Lupron to wind down or 'downregulate' the function of the ovary and so reduce production of oestrogen. HMG injections are then given to increase hormone levels.

Side effects: Similar to Clomid but primarily they include hot flushes, tiredness and, occasionally, headaches.

Human Menopausal Gonadotrophin (HMG):

This hormone is given by injection into the thigh or buttock. It is a means of providing the hormones FSH and LH (Follicle Stimulating Hormone and Luteinizing Hormone) which the pituitary gland also produces. Usually it is used in conjunction with Clomid or Buserelin.

Because the ovary is being stimulated artificially, over-stimulation is more likely, so that the drug should be administered only in an environment where ultrasound scan can be used to assess the risk of multiple birth.

Pure forms of pituitary gonadotrophins may be used (such as pure FSH) and these are used alone or in combination with HMG.

Side effects: Localised muscle tenderness, skin redness, fluid retention, headache, irritability, tiredness and depression, bloated feeling and abdominal pain. In exceptional cases, the pain and bloating may last 1-2 weeks.

Human Chorionic Gonadotrophin (HCG):

This hormone initiates the action of the hormone LH (Luteinizing Hormone) which is necessary to mature the egg and release it from the ovary.

It is often used in conjunction with Clomid, HMG or pure forms of FSH to effect ovulation. When this injection is given, it is expected that the egg will be released 36-38 hours later, so that it might be accompanied with advice on the timing of intercourse.

Side effects: Localised muscle tenderness.

Luteal Phase Support:

HCG is also used in smaller amounts at regular intervals to stimulate the ovary to produce progesterone after ovulation. It is always required in women using Buserelin or Lupron as the natural production of LH is supressed.

Progesterone helps change to occur in the endometrium necessary for implantation and subsequent pregnancy and may be used as an alternative or addition to LH hormone.

Side effects: Headache, irritability, restlessness, depression, fatigue, oedema and breast soreness.

Progesterone:

The hormone progesterone can be given directly either by injection (into the thigh or hip) or by pessaries administered vaginally or as a rectal suppository.

Side effects: Breast soreness, nausea and abdominal bloating.

Metrodin:

This is mainly FSH and has replaced HMG in many centres as it does not stimulate progesterone production and has little LH which is contained in HMG.

Gonadotrophin Releasing Hormone (GnRH):

This hormone is usually secreted by the base of the brain and stimulates or 'releases' the pituitary hormones FSH/LH in women, and testosterone in men. It is usually secreted in small amounts at regular intervals of about 16 times per day.

Injections of this hormone then need to be at frequent, regular intervals and therefore is best administered by a small battery-powered pump. It is not often used in IVF programs but is the drug of choice for women whose hypothalamus does not trigger pituitary hormone release.

A small needle is placed just under the skin of the abdomen and taped so it will not move. The pump is then attached and worn by the man or woman until ovulation or sperm production takes place.

Side effects: Abdominal discomfort, nausea, headache, backache, fatigue and breast soreness.

8
AND BABY MAKES THREE, OR FOUR...

The chance of becoming pregnant following treatment depends on the treatment carried out.

For the IVF procedure the pregnancy rate varies from as low as 8 per cent to 25 per cent for each treatment. The most common result is about 15 per cent. Patients who are older, those who have active endometriosis, those with only one ovary, or those who have more than one factor causing infertility may have lower rates. The remaining patients who are under 35 and have tubal disease, for example, would have a success rate of at least 20%. Women over 40 would have the lowest per cent chance, only 7 per cent per treatment.

The GIFT procedure has about twice the success rate of IVF, because the sperm and eggs are fertilised and grow in the tube and the laboratory media has not been able to duplicate that environment. Figures for the Australian clinics range from as low as 20 per cent to 40 per cent, the average being 30 per cent. Again, age does affect the success rate, for example, women over 40 have a success rate of 15 per cent.

There are other factors once the treatment has started which may affect the success rate. About one in 10 patients will not get to egg pickup although this dropout rate has diminished more recently since the clinics have been using the GnRH agonists like Buserelin and Lupron.

In a very small number of patients, no eggs are collected at the time of pickup. In women who have no eggs collected, there is either a very small number of ripe follicles and it is not possible for the doctor to collect eggs, or alternatively, there is a large number of follicles, but the follicles have not properly ripened.

In a small group of patients, the eggs will not fertilise when put with the sperm. When the eggs do not fertilise, there are two possible problems. There may be something wrong with the sperm quantity or quality. In the others, the egg quality is not good, the egg being unripe or structurally defective. The problem may be overcome in further treatments either by changing the method of stimulation of egg development or changing the method of preparation of the sperm.

Even if there is no obvious cause for the failure of fertilisation, the same result does not necessarily occur in a future treatment cycle, and it is often worth repeating the treatment at least once.

Couples often wonder how many treatments to pursue. In order to have a good chance of having a baby, one has to subtract one quarter from the pregnancy rate to obtain the take-home baby rate. This figure then has to be multiplied by the number of treatments to determine what is the likely chance of having a baby. Patients are advised to have at least five IVF attempts to have more than a 50 per cent chance of having a baby and for GIFT, four attempts gives you a 65 per cent chance of having a baby.

The success rate for each treatment is similar up to six treatments in most programs. Some women pursue up to 12 or more treatments in attempts to have a baby. The factors most likely to determine how many treatments a woman has are the costs (about $300 out of pocket expense per treatment), the stress, the social dislocation and emotional reaction to failure.

The major factor determining the success rate of these treatments is the number of eggs collected and, as a consequence, the number of embryos developed. In women who have only one embryo in IVF, the success rate has been around 7-8 per cent whereas it is about 15 per cent where there are two embryos, and 23 per cent with 3 or more.

In the GIFT procedure, the success rate is around 20 per cent with only one egg, rising to 30 per cent or more when there are three or more eggs collected.

Pregnancy will be confirmed by blood test done around the expected time of the patient's period, and the level of these hormones will also give some indication of whether the pregnancy is likely to be successful or not. The pregnancy is monitored by weekly blood tests, to check on oestrogen and progestogen levels and HCG (Human Chorionic Gonadotrophin). Nearly all women who suffer miscarriages or ectopic pregnancies have lower levels of one or more of these hormones. If hormone levels are low, an ultrasound done at 5½-6 weeks is done to determine whether there is a normal intrauterine pregnancy.

Ultrasounds are normally performed at around eight weeks of pregnancy, and blood tests are usually performed weekly up to this time. A patient who is likely to have a miscarriage will have this possibility discussed with her doctor. The earlier knowledge of miscarriage is helpful to most women, as it shortens the period of a pregnancy which is destined to failure. Once this is known, a termination can be performed to save several weeks of carrying a dead foetus.

Miscarriage is more common, occurring in about 20 per cent of IVF and GIFT pregnancies, the national figure being 13 per cent. One reason for this is the increased age of patients, as miscarriage is twice as common in women at 40 (26 per cent) as in women aged 25 (12 per cent). However, there may be other factors associated with the techniques that could also contribute to the miscarriage rate.

Women of 40 or more, having IVF, have a miscarriage rate of 40 per cent. Not only do they have a low chance of becoming pregnant, they also have a high chance of losing the pregnancy. The most likely explanation is the poorer quality of eggs in older women.

Ectopic pregnancy (pregnancy in the tube) occurs in 1 in 20 IVF and GIFT pregnancies. This is surprising in the case of IVF as the process bypasses the tubes. Although the embryo is confirmed by ultrasound to be placed in the uterus, the embryo later moves into the tube from the uterus. The reason for the high rate may be mostly related to patient problems.

Most ectopic pregnancies are detected by the eighth week of pregnancy. They are mostly treated by surgical intervention where the ectopic pregnancy is removed and the tube is conserved. When the tube is more severely damaged, part of the tube has to be removed. In many cases ectopic pregnancies can be dealt with by laparoscopy.

Another method of dealing with ectopic pregnancy is to inject a chemical into the sac to kill the pregnancy using ultrasound guidance, without having surgery. This is still an experimental technique which has possibilities as no surgical intervention is required.

In women who have severe tubal disease, it is preferable to have the inner tubes clipped prior to attempting IVF, as the risk of an ectopic pregnancy is double that of other IVF patients, about 10 per cent. This could be performed at the time of diagnostic laparoscopy.

TREATMENT DURING PREGNANCY

Most patients from IVF or GIFT are cared for by specialists who are familiar with the new technology. There is an increased risk of premature labour which is mostly related to the higher risk of multiple pregnancy, but even in women with a single pregnancy there is a 9 per cent chance of premature labour.

The use of hyperstimulation to produce more than one egg has resulted in about 20 per cent of the pregnancies being multiple, 17 per cent being twins and 3 per cent triplets. Very occasionally quadruplets and quintuplets have been reported. Most couples are pleased with the occurrence of twins as if they are over 35, they may have little chance of a further conception, and twins also avoid the need to come back on the program. The outcome for twins is very good. Although labour on average commences three weeks earlier, the degree of prematurity is usually not severe enough to be a hazard to the babies.

With triplets, the length of pregnancy on average is only 33 weeks, and with quadruplets about 28. These pregnancies are often associated with severe prematurity when there may be considerable hazards for the babies, not only of dying but surviving with mental or physical defect. When prematurity is severe and the baby weighs less than 1500gms, the risk of residual mental, physical and emotional defects is considerably higher. While it is an acceptable concept for some couples to have an immediate family of three children, it is not worth taking this risk because of the possibility of having a mentally or physically defective child. For these reasons, most programs are now reducing the number of embryos or eggs transferred in the procedures.

For the GIFT procedure, the number of eggs transferred has been gradually reduced from six to three in the Monash program, without significant reduction in the pregnancy rate. This has happened, we believe, because we can choose the best of the eggs collected so that if a woman produces 10 eggs, as long as we transfer the best three we will still have a relatively high pregnancy rate (30 per cent). This certainly excludes quadruplets but triplets have still occurred and we are now trying to transfer the two best eggs to see if we can exclude triplets but sustain a good pregnancy rate. So far the two egg GIFT has been successful.

In the case of IVF, the Australian programs have reduced the number of embryos transferred from four to three. However, if there are three good embryos transferred, there is still considerable risk of twins and triplets, and in these circumstances, when there are three good embryos, the patient should be warned of the risk of triplets and she can opt to have two transferred and the other good embryo frozen.

One other option in overseas centres still is to transfer large numbers of eggs and embryo but to offer patients selective termination, whereby unwanted foetuses are killed and the patient is left with the desired number of foetuses. The disadvantage of selective termination is the irony of creating human life and then partially killing it. Some religious groups would see selective abortion as unacceptable.

There is no reason why some patients who are pregnant cannot have normal deliveries, but there are factors mitigating against this—the increased age of the patient, the anxiety of both the patient and the obstetrician concerned, and the increased risks of premature delivery and multiple pregnancy. Twins and triplets may require caesarean section to protect the health of the foetus, and in some women the disease that has caused the infertility may also adversely influence the outcome of the pregnancy. For example, previous tubal surgery may increase the risk of rupture of the uterus during pregnancy.

For these reasons, the caesarean section rate in most programs is around 40 per cent. Caesarean section under local anaesthetic is now common, and does allow the woman to participate to some extent in the delivery.

Perinatal mortality is increased in both IVF and GIFT. This is mainly related to the increased risk of multiple pregnancies and prematurity, and the increased age of patients.

The risks of malformations is no higher than the general population, 2 per cent. However, the risk of several uncommon malformations, spina bifida, oesophageal atresia and urogenital malformation is more common.

There are precautions taken to diagnose spina bifida, with a vaginal ultrasound being carried out at 12 and 18 weeks. The problem with oesophageal atresia and urogenital malformations mostly can be overcome by surgery after birth.

9
MYTHS AND MISCONCEPTIONS

In this chapter we will look at the common myths and misconceptions that many readers probably have already encountered. Some will make you laugh; others will hurt.

How these myths begin is unimportant. How they gain credence and acceptance in the community shows that there is still a great deal of ignorance and a need for more education and public awareness about infertility.

Many couples expect to conceive within one or two months of attempting conception. It should be remembered that on average, it takes a healthy young couple having regular intercourse five cycles to get pregnant. If couples know and understand this, it saves them a lot of anxiety and expectation.

Approximately 10-15 per cent will not conceive in that first year of unprotected intercourse. At that stage, we feel it is time to start investigating the matter and try to pinpoint any problem.

One of the most common myths in human conception is that people get pregnant in two or three cycles. This does not happen with humans. This also allays the myth that women are at their most fertile during the first cycle off the contraceptive Pill.

Many couples also are under the impression that the position in which you have sexual intercourse may be important to conception. This can simply be labelled a myth.

MYTH: Infertility is primarily a woman's problem.

FACT: Possibly the most influential myth about infertility or childlessness is that it is a woman's problem and a man cannot be in any way 'at fault'. This is socially legitimated where there are severe social penalties for any man who admits that he has failed to make his partner pregnant.

In some societies, traditional folklore may make it unthinkable that anyone should believe a man could be responsible for his wife's failing to produce a child. In some parts of the world even giving birth to a girl is a cause of shame to a woman and she may be forced to produce babies year after year until she has given birth to a boy. Only then can she be regarded as a full member of her society and be allowed a rest from the bearing of children.

Where there is a lack of education, it is possible that the link between sexual intercourse and pregnancy is not preceived. One does not always need to look as far as an exotic tribe to find evidence of this ignorance.

Where the social status of a man is considered higher than that of a woman, it would be counter-productive for men to admit to something that would lower their own status in the eyes of other men if the blame could be legitimately shifted onto the woman.

Sometimes this shifting of 'blame' is a result of traditional acceptance of the very different roles assigned to men and women within a particular social group. From time to time, letters are received from women who cannot proceed with fertility investigations because their partner refuses to undertake any tests, or even in some cases, to accompany the woman to the hospital or clinic.

Thankfully, many men today do understand the need for semen analysis as a logical step in the infertility investigations.

Men do find it difficult to cope with the testing, sometimes, because they see this as an attack on their masculinity.

Unfortunately I still come across husbands who want their wives to go through all possible tests before they will even consider undergoing semen analysis. I find that frustrating because the semen analysis is the easiest test of all to do—with the exception of the temperature chart.

Would I agree to carry out all the investigations on the wife before doing a semen analysis on the husband? Only when the wife agrees to it. Some women say to me: "Do all the tests on me and then if you don't find anything, speak to my husband".

These women may need the medical support to speak to their partner to explain why he needs to undergo a semen analysis and a reminder that about 33 per cent of male partners are the main cause of infertility.

Not surprisingly, figures show that the problem is just as likely to lie with the man as the woman. There is also a third category of infertility where both partners are involved.

MYTH: The position for intercourse is important in achieving a pregnancy.

FACT: I know couples who believe they should assume certain positions after orgasm to ensure the sperm stays inside the vagina. Again, this is purely a myth.

One patient recently said her husband suspended her from five pillows so that she was almost vertical. We may all smile about this but it is easy to see why couples believe it is important for the sperm to remain inside the vagina for as long as possible. And in the case of the woman mentioned, she did get pregnant on the next cycle after resuming a more comfortable coital position.

As soon as the sperm leaves the penis they move quickly into the cervix and from here a few go straight into the fallopian tube within five minutes. A pool of sperm does remain in the cervix and will gradually move over the next 24 hours. But those that are left in the vagina do not do very well because it is an acidic environment. We find that the semen pool left in the vagina is unimportant in terms of getting pregnant. That is why spillage after intercourse is not important.

My advice to patients then is not to worry about positions for sexual intercourse—the sperm usually makes its way to the cervix anyway!

MYTH: The frequency of intercourse is important for getting pregnant more easily.

FACT: I know many couples who believe the sperm should be 'saved up' for the first two weeks of the cycle so that it is 'strong' and in good supply when ovulation is expected.

I think it is safe to say that in a healthy fertile male, it is not necessary to delay intercourse. With those men who may be borderline on a low sperm count, it is a good idea to abstain for two or three days prior to ovulation.

It is certainly true that abstinence may, for some men, be more deleterious. But the concept of saving up is not valid - certainly not beyond a couple of days.

So how often should you have intercourse during your ovulation cycle?

Firstly, try to define your fertile phase which is done by either studying temperature or mucous charts. Usually, a woman will ovulate between days 12-16 or 10-18. Once your phase is pinpointed, it is best to try to have intercourse every second day. Daily urine tests of the hormone LH will pinpoint ovulation accurately. The advantage of this is that it helps to alleviate a lot of anxiety trying to pick a specific day.

MYTH: Childless couples are as they are because of their psychological make-up.

FACT: They observe individual childless couples in states of distress or depression and assume this is the cause, rather than the result, of infertility. Another myth is that adoption increases fertility. Occasionally emotional changes lead to failure of ovulation or infrequent coitus, obvious causes of infertility.

At a more mundane level, those who have children may be totally unable to comprehend the reaction to their children from those who are not able to have children of their own.

When a childless person has to withdraw from all contacts with children as a safeguard against exposure to too much emotional stress, this is taken to mean that the childless are peculiar in some way. As the childless seem to have so little in common with others in normal social interaction and group membership, people find it hard to think of them as normal members of society.

And this is perhaps the most cruel myth of all.

MYTH: Infertility is incurable.

FACT: One myth which, fortunately, is slowly dying out, is that infertility is incurable. In the face of medical evidence to the contrary, it is surprising that this myth still holds ground. About 80 per cent of couples seeking treatment for infertility succeed. But it seems characteristic of many people that they build up their world picture from an amalgam of the experiences of those they come into contact with, and ideas they have inherited from family and childhood experiences.

Three or four cases of an event or occurrence are often sufficient for them to form a generalisation of potentially enormous magnitude. Statistical evidence cannot compete with this first-hand experience. Due to the difficulties involved for many people in obtaining satisfactory medical treatment for infertility, it is unfortunately possible for people to genuinely believe that infertility is incurable. The local hospital may have a very poor record, as a result of the lack of facilities for fertility treatments, or a low level of interest in the related fields of treatment.

Or a couple may decide to stop treatment, leaving friends convinced that here is another example of the incurability of infertility. The stress brought about by treatments can also lead to depression and a loss of interest in the sexual side of the relationship, thus perpetuating the likelihood of childlessness.

In the absence of a social climate which favours open discussion about fertility, it is difficult for most people to judge correctly, from observation of the experience of others, whether infertility can be 'cured' or not. Conversely, those people who keep quiet about their own medical investigations, and then, say, have a child by donor insemination, may never have to reveal that there is or was an infertility problem. It is hoped that exposure of the subject in the media will cause this myth to die out altogether in the not-too-distant future.

Some misconceptions about childlessness

Over the past few years there has developed a growing awareness, particularly but not exclusively, among younger people with a fairly high level of education, that the world is going through a crisis of a kind that humankind has never experienced before. Two particularly worrying features of the current world crisis are the enormous population increases likely before the end of the century, and the inequitable distribution and utilisation of the world's resources, particularly its irreplaceable resources.

The concentration on the necessity for population planning and control has, indirectly, had an adverse affect on the position of the involuntarily childless. As well as having to cope with the effects of widespread ignorance about their condition, they are increasingly being called upon to justify their decision to pursue lengthy or expensive fertility treatments in their quest to have their own child. It is somehow considered immoral or irresponsible of them to be so preoccupied with their own personal, even selfish, need for a child, when the world is so manifestly unable to provide adequately for the majority of the children it already has.

There are two answers to this. The first is that, despite the social problems caused by population increases, an individual does see his or her need for a child as personal, and of great importance. For most people, having a child is considered an essential and very much valued experience in life. Children are regarded as giving great pleasure, and they contribute to the quality of family life.

The second answer to the question as to whether the childless should be made to feel guilty for wanting a child in a overcrowded world is that, in pragmatic terms, the number of children likely to be born as a result of the pursuance of medical treatments will not have a perceptible influence on the population figures. It takes at least 2.3 children per family for a population to remain at the same level. The majority of the childless would want two children at the most. Many would be extremely satisfied with one child.

MYTH: Infertile couples are depriving others of medical care.

FACT: The childless are only 'depriving' others of treatment if the concept of a fixed health budget remains central in one's thinking. There are several areas of national spending which are quite controversial, for example, the defence budget, and in almost every country in the world this budget is a source of contention. The childless have to argue their case, not as attempting to deprive the sick of vital resources, but as demanding adequate consideration from the national budget as a whole.

Health budgets compensate many patients for illnesses where the patient is at fault, having been a heavy smoker or drinker, or a drug addict. In contrast, less than 20 per cent of infertile couples have contributed to their own problem.

10
A HELPING HAND

All patients entering our IVF program, as part of the pre-screening requirements, must attend at least one counselling session. Counselling sessions are a requirement of the law under the Infertility (Medical Procedures) Act of 1984. For some couples, the thought of attending a counselling session may be daunting, so we asked one of IMC's counsellors, Diane Molloy, to answer some questions which may help to allay any concerns.

Diane joined the centre in 1990 and has a background in Social Work. She also has undertaken post graduate study in Child Development, and Child and Family Therapy. Prior to commencing employment at IMC, Diane worked chiefly in the areas of Child and Family Psychiatry, Adoption Information Services, and as Co-ordinator of a Social Work Student Unit.

We asked Diane the following:

Q. *Why are counselling sessions necessary?*

A. It is a legal requirement that any couple (that is, both husband and wife) entering an IVF or related infertility program, or donating embryos or gametes must have at least one counselling session. The counselling is not an assessment, but an opportunity to talk in detail about the program, issues arising from infertility or treatment, or important decisions that may have to be made prior to starting the program. We are guided by what each couple want to know and discuss, and in how much detail. Although the minimum number of sessions is one, couples are encouraged to return for as many sessions as they feel are helpful.

The counsellors are also available for additional support during or between treatment cycles.

Q. *Are the counselling sessions in groups or for individual couples?*

A. Both group and individual sessions are an option. Couples can decide which would suit their needs.

Q. *If I have already been on an IVF cycle and had a counselling session a few years ago, do I need to have another session before starting the program again?*

A. If a couple have had their last IVF treatment more than 12 months ago we recommend another counselling session as an opportunity to update information about any major changes in treatment procedures. Couples have found these sessions useful to discuss difficulties, queries and concerns. The sessions are not mandatory; the choice remains with the couple.

Q. *What are some of the questions that you are asked most often?*

A. Questions vary considerably, often depending on the couple's understanding of their diagnosis and its relationship to their infertility, and what IVF treatment entails.

Many couples are still a little unsure about community acceptance of IVF and how parents and friends may respond to the couple's disclosure about their infertility, and to the infertility treatment, whether it be from the IVF program, the donor gamete program or a combination of both.

Questions may relate to issues such as who should the couple tell, how much information should they give, and when. Often there is concern about the impact of the treatment on the couple's relationship, and what can be done to minimise stress.

Questions commonly asked include: How can I be sure that my eggs will be fertilised with my husband's sperm? Can embryos get mixed up and transferred to the wrong couple? Are babies born from IVF procedures, especially frozen embryos, the same as normal babies?

No question is silly or stupid. Every couple has the right to information and knowledge and often asking questions and discussing information is the most potent means of reassurance and reducing anxiety and apprehension.

Q. *What sort of questions do you ask as a counsellor?*

A. I ask questions to help me understand each couple's case. For example, it is helpful to know how long they have been trying to conceive, a little about how their diagnosis has affected them, and what treatments they have had and also what their expectations are of IVF.

I also may ask whether couples have shared the knowledge of their infertility and treatment with friends or family. Discussing this can be helpful in terms of building support networks and helping couples get through the emotional highs and lows of treatment. For some couples, however, telling family and friends is more stressful and they may ask for help in establishing other methods of support. Alternative suggestions may include relaxation techniques, support from other couples on the program, self help groups or the staff at IMC. Literature or additional counselling can also be helpful.

It is important to remember that everyone is an individual, and their needs and how they can best be supported will vary.

Q. *Do couples using either donor sperm or donor eggs require counselling?*

A. Yes, legislation requires that recipients of donor gametes receive counselling.

Couples often use their counselling time as an opportunity to share concerns and discuss issues and decisions that are difficult to talk about with family and friends. Examples include: Whether the child should be told of his/her origins; how might the use of donor gametes affect the relationship between husband and wife; will the relationship between the child and the non genetic parent be different compared to children conceived by the parenting couple?

Sometimes, as the result of counselling, couples realise that they are not ready to start treatment, often because they have not yet resolved their grief for the child that they cannot have. Other couples find reassurance in the fact that their doubts and apprehensions are normal.

Q. *Is there a difference between recipients of donor eggs and donor sperm?*

A. There are differences between the treatments. The recipient of donor eggs is also the infertile partner in the couple. Although the wife does not genetically contribute to the child, she has an important physical role in carrying the pregnancy and giving birth, a process that significantly contributes to the bonding between the mother and the child. More over, the treatment is medically complex and involves many aspects of normal IVF treatment.

On the other hand, for a couple using Donor Insemination, the procedure is relatively simple and focused on the fertile partner. This can lead to the common experience of the husband feeling unimportant and left out, and maybe guilty because he is the infertile partner.

While there are shared issues and concerns by couples on the Donor Insemination Program and the Donor Egg Program, there are also intrinsically different issues and adjustments.

Q. *Do egg and sperm donors receive counselling?*

A. Yes, again legislation requires that the donor and his/her spouse, if the donor is married, must be given the same opportunities as the recipient, to know his/her rights and responsibilities and discuss any issues or queries. For donors who are giving to unknown recipients, it is a time to consider how they might feel about helping in the conception of a child/or children that they might never know. Whether they would tell future partners of their donation? How they might feel if in the future they could not have children of their own?

Men and women donating to known recipients are frequently faced with more complex issues, questions and decisions to consider than their counterparts donating to unknown recipients.

In a known situation, whilst there are no definitive answers, donors and recipients must remain open to many issues, such as how each person involved might feel about the donor having ongoing knowledge and/or contact with the child, and should the donor tell his/her own children a child is born as the result of the donation.

Although many women receiving IVF treatment have generously offered to donate excess eggs, a large proportion of the donated eggs currently used are from fertile women who have chosen to give to another. This necessarily involves follicle stimulation and surgery as with IVF treatment where the patient's own gametes are used. Unlike sperm donation, a woman wishing to donate eggs must also consider the physical discomfort that she may face, and the impact of treatment on her family and daily routine. At times this decision is made more difficult if the donor's husband is fearful for the health of his wife, or unsure about the implications of donation for himself and his family.

Counselling can assist in facilitating discussion between the couple to identify concerns, and often to rectify misconceptions. Counselling does not however, tell the couple what they ought to do, or make judgements as to who is right or wrong. These decisions remain at all times with the couple.

Q. *Do you see your role expanding?*

A. Our plans include making ourselves more available for counselling and support to couples at all stages of treatment, initiating workshops and seminars to raise community and fellow professionals' awareness of infertility, the issues it raises for couples and the impact it can have on families. Most importantly, we hope to open people's minds to the growing numbers of ways IVF treatment can help couples become families.

PATIENT REQUIREMENTS

Prior to starting any IVF treatment, couples are required to register at the IMC. At this time they will pay a small joining fee and will receive a registration letter outlining pre-screening requirements, a handbook and general consent forms, membership for Friends of IVF, and a Newsletter.

Pre-treatment screening requirements include blood tests for HIV (AIDS) and Hepatitis B (husband and wife), Rubella immunity and Sperm Antibodies (wife only), and ultrasound scan to assess the ovaries and uterus, and two semen analyses.

From time to time, additional information related to changes in procedures, new research projects or items of general interest may also be included.

It is recommended that you do not fill out any of the forms until you have read your handbook and seen the counsellor. Counselling allows you the opportunity to discuss any questions or concerns, and can assist you to make decisions required in the general consent, such as whether to freeze or not freeze embryos, selecting the maximum number of eggs/embryos for transfer, and whether to donate or dispose of excess eggs or embryos. Other specific consents may be required to be signed at counselling sessions, or prior to, or during treatment.

Many initial decisions, such as whether to donate embryos or not, can be changed with sufficient notice during the course of treatment, as couples may feel differently once they have actually experienced the program, or become pregnant.

The Patient Information Forms are designed to meet the requirements of the legislation that stipulates that all recipients and donors of donor gametes/embryos must register specific identifying and non-identifying information at the Health Department of Victoria. You will be given these to be filled out if you are considering or intend to donate embryos or gametes, or if you are a recipient of the same.

Throughout the treatment, additional written information will be given to all patients. If patients still have any queries they are encouraged to ask their clinicians or other appropriate staff members.

11
FACING FACTS

If you wanted to highlight the legal, ethical and emotional problems that have surrounded IVF in the past decade, three important cases need to be discussed.

First, the Rios story. This is a sad story of two people, Elsa and Mario Rios, who were based in Los Angeles. They came to Melbourne in 1980 hoping, like many couples, that IVF could provide them with a child.

Elsa had one attempt which failed and left two frozen embryos in storage for a later attempt. Unfortunately she never got a chance to have the frozen embryos implanted. Elsa and her husband were killed in a plane crash in 1983. What they left behind created a maze of complicated legal and ethical problems, some of which are still to be solved.

When she first approached the Melbourne team, Elsa was 40 and her husband 57. As the American IVF program was still in its infancy and, at that stage, still to achieve a successful pregnancy, they pleaded with the Melbourne team to allow them to try IVF in this country.

I have to say that the Rios case was one of the saddest I had heard about. They had lost their only daughter in a tragic accident in 1979. Then 10, Elsa's daughter from a previous marriage had accidentally shot and killed herself at the couple's home. Elsa never got over the accident and was determined they should have another child.

Investigations showed that Mario had a low sperm count and it seemed unlikely Elsa would be able to become pregnant by her husband.

They agreed to try fertilisation by donor sperm and three eggs were collected, two of which were frozen.

The couple returned to America to rest before trying a frozen cycle, but in 1983 both were killed in a plane accident.

At that time, IVF still had many legal 'loopholes' to be ironed out. One legal problem which this case highlighted was the fact that no decision had been made about what should happen to the frozen embryos in the case of death, or for that matter, divorce.

This is now mandatory of course and explains why we ask all potential patients to sign a form determining what would happen to any frozen embryos in the event of death or divorce.

EMBRYO DONATION

The choices you now have include donation to another couple for the purposes of implantation or for use in legally permitted research and experimentation, donation to another couple only for implantation; donation for use of legally permitted research and experimentation only; or to allow the embryos to be disposed of.

You and your husband must make a decision before actually starting any IVF treatment.

The Rios case set in motion lengthy legal and moral debate and authorities had to make a decision about the fate of the embryos. In 1984, the chairman of a state government appointed ethics committee, Professor Louis Waller, said the Rios embryos should be allowed to die with dignity.

That same year, the Infertility (Medical Procedures) Act was passed. It was amended in 1988 and is expected to be reviewed again. The Act allowed for the embryos to be donated to another couple. But this in turn raised the question of whether an infertile couple should be allowed to 'adopt' the Rios embryos.

If this was allowed, would the embryos have a claim to the substantial estate left behind by Mario and Elsa Rios? Other options discussed in 1984 included the use of the embryos for experimentation or the disposal of the embryos.

In 1988, the Victorian Crown Solicitor's office recommended that the embryos be made available to another infertile couple.

Sadly, it was then discovered that no AIDS test had been carried out on the mother nor the sperm donor. It is now law that all couples involved in any IVF procedures (both as recipients or as donors) must first undertake an AIDS test.

Because the mother and donor in the Rios case had not had this test, it effectively meant that they could never have been made available to another couple for 'adoption'.

The Victorian Health Minister must now decide the fate of the Rios embryos—a decision expected to be announced when the Infertility (Medical Procedures) Act is reviewed.

This Act gives the Minister for Health power to decide on the uses of the frozen embryos that cannot be implanted because of death or injury to the patient.

Ironically, I doubt whether the Rios embryos would actually survive the thawing process anyway. The preservation techniques used in 1981 are not as advanced as those in use now.

CUSTODY BATTLE

Another case which put the Victorian IVF program under close scrutiny was that of a young Gippsland couple who took their custody battle over seven frozen embryos to the Family Court in 1989. The couple had separated and had seven frozen embryos in storage at a Melbourne hospital.

Sadly, the woman had miscarried triplets five months into a pregnancy the year before and the couple cited this, along with other marital problems, as the cause of the breakdown of their marriage.

The husband withdrew his consent to allow his estranged wife to implant the embryos and this led to one of the country's first custody battles over embryos.

This case really voiced a common concern of many men on IVF programs. The husband in this case was reportedly worried about his financial responsibilities should his estranged wife become pregnant with the frozen embryos.

Many of the husbands involved in IVF have similar concerns. What this case did was to highlight the need for open, realistic discussion about what would happen to frozen embryos in the event of divorce.

The law as it stands makes it clear that couples on IVF programs must be married. If you have embryos frozen and divorce, then, according to Victorian law, you don't have access to those embryos.

But I find it hard to imagine that the state would confiscate or dispose of somebody's embryos because they have been divorced. I think if this were ever to happen, they would face a lot of public opposition from all sorts of groups.

Let's face it, in our society we make provisions for the children from divorced couples. Surely potential children should have the same considerations and should be allocated to the most appropriate of the parents. Perhaps in the future, a legal document could be drawn up releasing the husband from financial responsibilities to allay any fears he may have. At present though, the law does not allow a husband to document himself out of paying maintenance for children. This custody battle had repercussions for many of the 3000 couples currently on IVF programs in Victoria.

It forced into the limelight the legal document all couples are required to sign - a contract that says what will happen to the frozen embryos in the event of death or divorce.

When the Victorian Government's IVF committee thrashed out legal and ethical problems, the question of custody to one parent or the other could not be addressed because, legally, IVF is only for married couples.

The couple mentioned here are obviously not the first to separate and have frozen eggs in storage. In other cases, the couples agreed to dispose of the embryos so there wasn't a legal or moral problem. But I think what this case did do was to force couples to think more carefully about the options. I appreciate it is difficult for couples to have to think about what would happen if they divorce because they are on the verge of trying to create a family usually after much heartbreak and years of trying to conceive on their own. I do try to bring the issue up with couples because I believe it is something they have to consider and discuss. In the case we have been discussing, the couple settled out of court and agreed to donate the frozen embryos to infertile couples.

The issue of donation is important and has been dealt with quite well in the Infertility (Medical Procedures) Act, 1984. I believe it is innovative because in Victoria, by law, the infertile couple are the legal parents. Many people are not aware of this fact because of the many stories they read from overseas regarding disputes over custody where a surrogate mother has been used. This is one of the issues that frightens many couples about using donor sperm or eggs. It should also be pointed out that the donor has no claims on the child at all. The child also has no claims on the donor.

SURROGACY

Surrogacy is another important issue awaiting a review of the Infertility (Medical Procedures) Act.

A recent case to highlight how important this issue is to many couples is that of two Sydney sisters. The fertile sister, Deborah, wants to have her younger sister's baby. The younger sister, Bronwyn, was diagnosed in 1982 as having cancer and is now in remission. A pregnancy, however, would put her life in jeopardy and surrogacy is her only option to have a child. The sisters and their husbands, like several other couples in this country, have been in a legal limbo for four years waiting for a review of the Act to allow altruistic IVF surrogacy. The sisters believe that time is running out for them.

Bronwyn and her husband Craig say when they married in 1985 they knew children were out of the question because of Bronwyn's medical background. They were warned that the volatile hormone cocktail that pregnancy produces could trigger the cancer again. Adoption too was out of the question because of her condition. The couple decided it was best for Bronwyn to have her fallopian tubes tied to prevent pregnancy.

But her sister never gave up hope of Bronwyn and Craig having the child they wanted. She read an article on surrogacy and discussed an idea with her husband, Iain. They then told Bronwyn and Craig that Deborah was prepared to act as a surrogate for her sister. In Deborah's words: "Bronwyn deserves to be a mother. She is really fantastic with children and I think she should have a chance at this." Bronwyn—a qualified midwife—actually delivered her sister's last baby.

Australia's first—and to date only—successful surrogacy was in 1988 when Victorian sisters Maggie and Linda Kirkman co-produced baby Alice. After Alice's birth, all other IVF surrogacy in Victoria was put on hold because the Infertility (Medical Procedures) Act then prevented Professor John Leeton and his team carrying on with the work. Professor Leeton said the main problem was that IVF was technically meant only for infertile couples. This is frustrating to Professor Leeton and his team because he has at least a dozen couples ready and waiting. He believes the current surrogacy laws in Victoria are discriminatory and should not stop couples going ahead with their plans.

In Victoria, Section 13 of the Infertility (Medical Procedures) Act of 1984 outlaws a fertile mother being implanted with an embryo if she is capable of becoming pregnant.

Maggie Kirkman said words failed her when told of the plight of Bronwyn and her sister Deborah. The genetic mother of Australia's first IVF surrogate baby said she could imagine how the women felt. "It would be a mixture of anger, despair and yearning," Maggie said. "The critics talk about exploitation. Well I know from our experience that no one in our family was exploited."

Maggie had a hysterectomy more than a decade ago and her husband Severn was infertile. Her younger sister, Linda, agreed to become a surrogate and Alice was born in Melbourne in 1988.

That sounds simple but Maggie said it took them two years to convince Professor Leeton to go ahead with the procedure.

She added she felt for Bronwyn and Deborah because she knew how heartbreaking it was to know the technology was available, to know they could have a child, but the law was preventing it.

EMBRYO EXPERIMENTATION

Embryo experimentation is prohibited in Victoria except under special circumstances. Embryo experimentation was required to determine the safety of IVF. Embryos were checked for chromosomal damage before the technique was used to transfer IVF embryos to patients.

Experimentation may help develop new infertility treatments and determine some of the causes of congenital malformations. It may also help us understand how organs develop and function, thus assisting in the understanding and treatment of adult diseases.

The Victorian committee has agreed to allow the studying of embryos to determine the safety of new infertility techniques. This was done before microinjection of sperm was used to help men with severe infertility problems. Normal pregnancies have now resulted from this technique.

Embryo biopsy has been developed to sex embryos. This is not harmful to the embryo and allows couples with sex-linked diseases, such as haemophilia, to avoid tests done later in pregnancy and subsequently the possible need for therapeutic abortion. Embryos of the sex which carry the disease can be discarded, while embryos free of the disease can be transferred to the patient.

Embryo biopsy can also be used for genetic testing of embryos. Genetic testing for cystic fibrosis, thalassaemia and other diseases may soon be available. Only a single cell of the embryo is required for the test and the embryo is not affected by the biopsy. The chance of pregnancy and a normal child is not altered by the biopsy. There are ethical advantages in preferring embryo biopsy and IVF to natural conception and the possibility of abortion. The main disadvantage is that the woman undergoes IVF and may not succeed in becoming pregnant unless she undergoes many attempts.

Using embryos for research which kills the embryo is not accepted by some people on various grounds: the sanctity of life, the potential of the embryo to form a human being, and the moral status of the embryo. Opponents of this view claim that the early embryo has diminished moral status because of its biological status, lacks personal qualities, and is unable to feel, think or be conscious. They also cite the scant regard by the community who use IUDs for contraception and are not concerned by early embryo death when there is no missed period.

12
ANSWERING THE CRITICS

Since the birth of Australia's first In Vitro Fertilisation baby, Candice Reid, back in 1981, IVF has attracted much media attention both in Australia and around the world.

Some of this has been positive, but all too often reports have focused on the negative aspects of the program.

I understand how alarming it can be for an IVF patient and her family to read reports which are highly critical of the program—from the drugs we use to stimulate ovulation to advances in technology such as embryo freezing and embryo experimentation.

In this chapter I want to look at some of these negative media reports and discuss the issues they raise.

I find it is easier to do this by answering some of the questions IVF patients have raised on this issue in past years.

Q. *An article in 'Choice' magazine claimed that IVF couples risked exploitation and that some clinics, intentionally or not, used subtle forms of persuasion to pressure women into potentially risky procedures. Is this true?*

A. Any couple can be exploited if insufficient information is given to them. The magazine researched 18 IVF clinics to see whether they were "fully informing prospective patients about the levels of success and risks associated with IVF technology and treatment." The 'Choice' article also mentioned that some clinics including IMC, go to a great deal of effort to inform patients adequately.

I hope that all clinics always endeavour to inform patients

adequately of all risks and levels of success. We aim to give our patients honest, realistic information so the choice about IVF can be their own.

Q. *The article also claimed that the 'potentially risky procedures included the implantation of four or more embryos, which raises the chances of multiple pregnancy'.*

A. As mentioned throughout this book and as mentioned to all our patients, we have decreased the number of eggs and embryos transplanted to reduce the risk of multiple pregnancy.

We do not encourage patients to have 'four or more embryos' transplanted. In fact the maximum number of embryos we allow to be transplanted on IVF is now three (unless the patient is over 40 years).

But again I stress that the decision on the number of embryos transferred is entirely a decision of the couple involved. I would not like to think patients are being pressured in any way to risk a multiple pregnancy.

Q. *That article also said that IVF doctors are well paid. Is that true?*

A. Yes, it is true we are well paid but no more than other specialist physicians. The Infertility Medical Centre has returned profits to research in the cause and treatment of infertility.

Q. *I was concerned about an article in 'The Lancet' which said IVF is associated with serious health risks. What risks was the article referring to?*

A. 'The Lancet' said IVF was associated with serious health risks to babies born on the program, and also possibly to their mothers. It went on to say that because of the problems associated with IVF, clinics should require special accreditation and be constantly monitored.

It added that IVF was expensive and benefited only a small portion of infertile couples.

The risk of baby death at and soon after birth is higher than normal conceptions, about 2 to 3 per 100 births. This is mainly due to the increased age of patients and multiple pregnancies, where prematurity increases the risks at and soon after birth. As 97-98/100 babies are liveborn and risks are consistent with other obstetric factors there is no special need for concern. All pregnant women after IVF or GIFT are cared for by specialist obstetricians.

A study of 14,000 IVF babies shows no increase in risk of congenital abnormalities.

IVF is not expensive compared with other high technology procedures such as heart and kidney treatments. The cost per baby is about $30,000 for IVF and $18,000 for GIFT. Because the Government and private health insurance agencies subsidise treatments, the out of pocket costs per treatment are only $350. In Australia over 5,000 babies have been born following IVF and GIFT. Technology derived from these treatments has helped several thousand other infertile women to become pregnant. IVF and GIFT are only required when simpler treatments fail.

The risk to the patient is very small. In over 10,000 treatments at the IMC only two women have required surgery subsequently for infection or bleeding.

Q. *What is happening with embryo experimentation?*

A. It was reported in November, 1990, that the Victorian Government had temporarily halted embryo experimentation because of community concern.

The Standing Review and Advisory Committee on Infertility was asked by the (then) Minister for Health, Mrs Hogg, to defer further investigations by scientists for embryo experimentation until after its report had been considered by parliament and the community.

There has been plenty of debate within the community over embryo experimentation. At present, under existing legislation, experiments on unborn human life are limited to embryos no older than 22 hours.

In 1989, the committee was asked to review embryo experimentation after public debate about the legality of such experiments and a moratorium was placed on experiments.

This was lifted in May, 1990, after the Government received the first part of the report. The committee acknowledged that it had the power to approve post-syngamy experiments on embryos. Syngamy is the stage at which the chromosomes of an egg and sperm come together.

The second part of the committee's report was to be tabled

late in 1990 and the Minister at the time said there were parts of the Infertility (Medical Procedures) Act, 1984, which required further examination.

Q. *Why is embryo experimentation important?*

A. It is a vital part of infertility research, helping to find causes and new treatments. One important example is that it would allow scientists to detect sex-linked genetic diseases from a single cell. This will not harm the embryo. This has the obvious advantage of stopping those carriers of sex-linked genetic diseases from passing them on.

Embryo experiments allow scientists to find out more about the cause of abnormalities in babies by studying how things go wrong in the earliest stages of man's development.

Q. *The National Bioethics Consultative Committee has recommended that a national code on reproductive technology be introduced for people born as a result of sperm, ovum or embryo donation. What other recommendations of the committee are being considered?*

A. The National Bioethics Consultative Committee (NBCC) has been investigating a number of issues raised as a consequence of IVF and related procedures since May, 1988.

In particular, it is looking at the issue of surrogacy, which it said in the first part of the report (released mid-1990) was of great social, legal and ethical significance. It has recommended that surrogacy may be allowed on a non-commercial basis, providing there was control over the procedures and counselling for those involved.

As part of its investigations into surrogacy, the NBCC proposed a national code on reproductive technology so that all children born as a result of donated sperm, ovum or embryo could, in future, get information about the donor and donors could have the right to find out about any children they helped produce.

The committee has recommended that when couples and donors wanted to enter a program, consent to rules on getting information about a child at a later date would be a pre-condition.

Q. *I have read stories quoting Dr Renate Klein where she says women should abandon IVF because it is medically unethical* *and puts the health of women at risk. What are your comments?*

A. Dr Klein has also criticised IVF because she says the program ignores the physical and financial cost to women.

The physical risks of IVF are extremely low. In over 10,000 treatments at the Infertility Medical Centre there have been no deaths, and no serious illness resulting from the procedure. Bleeding and infection—complications of nearly every surgical technique—is very uncommon. Side effects during drug treatment are the commonest problems—tiredness and abdominal discomfort being most common. There is no known risk of permanent ill health, including cancer. The cost for each treatment is only $350 if the patient has private health insurance.

Q. *I have read various articles about cloning. What is it and will it ever be possible in Australia?*

A. Cloning refers to the making of replicas. This can be achieved in the embryo by splitting the embryo. This is useful in veterinary industry to increase reproductive efficiency by making artificial twins. It has not been accepted as a procedure for infertile patients. Replicas of adults are not possible.

Q. *I have read that the Infertility (Medical Procedures) Act is currently under review. Are there any sections of this Act you would like to see changed?*

A. Yes. The Act served a good purpose in producing guidelines for the practice of a new technology. However, Statutes are rigid and were made at a time when neither the community nor those involved in IVF were well enough informed to appreciate the disadvantages of the Act.

IVF is an accepted medical procedure throughout the world with few medical and social problems when IVF involves couples using their own sperm and eggs. Its practice in this form should not be restricted, does not need Government control to decide who should have the procedure and where it should be done, does not need compulsory counselling for the infertile couples, should be available to de facto couples, and information concerning the couples should not be available to the government authorities to peruse. The Victorian Government has two committees involved in this control, a waste of money for an impoverished State.

The Act should be retained for the use of donor gametes where the legislation has been imaginative and protective of the interests of the couples and future children.

The section on embryo experimentation is useless as its meaning is uncertain and it does not reflect community attitudes to the early embryo, which has no protection in law in relation to natural conception.

13
IVF SPEAK

Adhesion: The sticking of ovaries, tubes, uterus, bowel and abdominal lining to one or more of each other affecting fertility. May follow pelvic surgery, tubal infections or endometriosis.
AIH: Artificial Insemination Husband.
AIDS: Acquired Immune Deficiency Syndrome.
Amenorrhoea: The absence of menstruation for more than six months.
Amniocentesis Test: Fluid is removed from around the foetus and used to check for congenital abnormalities e.g. Down's syndrome.
Andrology: The study of male fertility and infertility.
Anovulation: An occasional or persistent failure to mature and release an egg. This is not necessarily the same as "amenorrhoea" as periods may occur with anovulation.
Antibody: In infertility, a compound in the blood, cervical mucous or semen which interferes with normal sperm function or fertilisation.
Aspermia: Absence of semen.
Azoospermia: Total lack of sperm.
Basal Temperature Chart: The daily measurement of the woman's temperature before getting out of bed each morning. The chart may show a rise in temperature in the second half of the cycle which suggests that ovulation has occurred.
Biopsy: A sample of living tissue taken for microscopic examination.
Boost//Flare: The use of hormones to firstly stimulate the ovary, and secondly to prevent natural ovulation - the hormones are similar to the natural gonadotrophic releasing hormones.
Bromocriptine: A drug effective in treating infertility due to a high prolactin hormonal level.

Capacitation: Change in sperm which is required before the sperm can fertilise the egg—metabolic and movement changes occur.
Catheter: A plastic tube which is used to carry eggs and sperm in the GIFT procedure or embryos when transferring embryos from the laboratory to the uterus in the IVF procedure.
Centrifuge: A process to separate substances of different specific gravity e.g. used to separate sperm from the fluid contained in the semen.
Cervical pH: A measurement of the acidity of the mucus in the cervix; if acidity is high it may affect sperm movement.
Cervix: The lower part of the uterus that connects with the vagina.
Chromosomes: Contain genes which are the chemical 'blue print' for all life. Each cell has a double set of identical chromosomes, in all 46. The reproductive cells, the sperm and egg, have a single set of chromosomes, 23 each, which combine to form an embryo containing 46 chromosomes. A special set of chromosomes, the X and Y, determine one's sex, XY being a male and XX a female.
Cilia: Microscopic hair-like projections from the surface of a cell capable of beating in a co-ordinated fashion. In the tube they move the embryo towards the uterus.
Clomiphene or Clomid: A drug to stimulate the ovary to produce follicles.
Coitus: Sexual relations.
Conception: The union between the sperm and the egg.
Corpus Luteum: The special gland that forms in the ovary at the site of ovulation and produces the hormone progesterone in the second half of the normal menstrual cycle.
Cryopreservation: Use of freezing to preserve embryos for future use - requires a chemical preservant.
Cysts: Fluid contained in sac - most common in ovary.
Dilatation and Curettage: (D & C) Dilatation of the cervix to allow scraping of the uterine lining with an instrument (curette). Can be done as a diagnostic measure in infertility.
DI: Artificial Insemination by donor semen.
Diathermy: An electric current used to damage tissue e.g. to close a blood vessel or remove abnormal tissue such as endometriosis.
Down Regulation: The ovary is suppressed by using gonadotrophic like releasing hormones (Lucrin) after which the ovary is stimulated by pituitary hormone (HMG).
Down's Syndrome: A chromosomal abnormality in the foetus which

may cause severe mental retardation, cardiac abnormalities and facial characteristics; it may be due to increased age of the mother, (>37 years) or run in the family.
Dysmenorrhoea: Painful menstruation.
Dyspareunia: Painful intercourse.
Ectopic Pregnancy: A pregnancy in which the fertilised egg implants anywhere but in the uterine cavity. This is usually in the fallopian tube.
Ejaculate: Semen ejected from the penis during orgasm.
Embryo: The earliest stage of human development - the 2 weeks from entry of the sperm into the egg until a multiple cell structure with a fluid sac inside is formed, called the blastocyst.
Endocrinologist: A doctor who specialises in diseases of the endocrine glands (glands producing hormones).
Endometrium: The lining of the uterus which grows and is shed each cycle.
Epididymis: A special duct at the back of the testes for the storage and further development of sperm as they mature.
ET (Embryo Transfer): A simple procedure where the embryos are placed inside the uterus by passing a fine catheter through the neck of the uterus.
Fallopian Tubes: a pair of narrow tubes that carry the egg from the ovary to the body of the uterus. Fertilisation occurs in the outer end of the tube.
Fertilisation: The penetration of the egg by the sperm.
Foetus: The foetus refers to a developing human being, between 2 weeks of development and birth.
Fibroids (Fibromyomata): A benign tumour of muscular tissue that occurs in the uterine wall. May be totally without symptoms or may cause abnormal menstrual patterns. They sometimes cause infertility.
Fimbriae: The fringed and flaring outer ends of the fallopian tubes which pick up the sticky egg from the ovary.
Follicle: The cells surrounding a developing egg in the ovary.
Follicle Stimulating Hormone (FSH): A hormone from the pituitary gland which is essential for the growth of ovarian follicles in the woman and sperm production in the man.
Gamete: The male or female reproductive cells, the sperm or the egg.
Genetic: Pertaining to hereditary characteristics dependent on action of chemicals called genes.

Gestation: The period of foetal development in the uterus from the conception to birth. In humans this is usually considered to be forty weeks from the last period.
Gift: Gamete Intra Fallopian Transfer.
Gonads: The glands that make the gametes, the testicles in the male and the ovaries in the female.
Haemorrhage: Excessive bleeding.
HMG: Human Menopausal Gonadotrophins contain two hormones, FSH and LH, which stimulate egg development and egg release (ovulation).
Hormone: A chemical produced by an endocrine gland in the body that circulates in the blood and has widespread action throughout the body.
Human Chorionic Gonadotrophin (HCG): A hormone secreted by the placenta in pregnancy that prolongs the life of the corpus luteum which in turn preserves the pregnancy. The presence of this hormone accounts for a positive pregnancy test. It may also be administered via injection to treat some infertility problems.
Humegon: Human pituitary gonadotrophin, used to stimulate egg development and ovulation.
Hydrocoele: A swelling in the scrotum containing fluid.
Hydrosalpinx: A serious cause of infertility where the tube is blocked at the ovarian end and contains clear fluid.
Hydrotubation: Flushing fluid through the tubes to check that they are open.
Hypothalamus: A small area at the base of the brain which is connected to and controls the pituitary gland. The latter releases FSH and LH under the direction of the hypothalamus.
Hysterectomy: The surgical removal of the uterus.
Hysterosalpingogram: An x-ray to see if the tubes are open. It also shows the internal outline of the uterus.
Hysteroscopy: Telescope placed through cervix inside uterus to detect abnormalities.
Idiopathic Infertility: Infertility of unknown cause, constituting 10 per cent of all infertile couples.
Implantation: The embedding of an embryo in the endometrium of the uterus.
Impotence: The inability of the male to achieve or maintain an erection for intercourse, due to physical or emotional problems or combined factors.

Incompetent Cervix: A weakened cervix that is incapable of holding the foetus within the uterus for 40 weeks, sometimes a cause of late miscarriage. May affect a pregnancy from sixteen weeks onwards.
Infertility: Inability to conceive, an arbitrary time of one year being accepted, as 90 per cent of couples conceive by this time.
Insemination: The process of placing sperm with eggs to attempt fertilisation.
Intra-Uterine Insemination (IUI): insertion of sperm into the uterus in order to achieve conception; sometimes used for unknown infertility, cervical mucous barrier and male infertility.
IUD (Intrauterine Device): A contraceptive consisting of plastic or metals, placed inside the uterus.
IVF—In Vitro Fertilisation: Fertilising and culturing of a human egg outside the body with the intention of introducing the embryo into the uterus.
Kremer Test: This determines whether the sperm or cervical mucous are responsible for sperm failing to pass through the cervix (neck of womb).
Laparoscopy: A surgical investigation using a telescope-like instrument to have a look at the pelvic organs.
Laparotomy: An abdominal incision to explore and treat a condition. Also used in abdominal surgery.
Lucrin: Gonadotrophin blocking hormone used to control ovary in stimulation cycle.
Luteal Phase: The last 11 - 17 days of a cycle following ovulation.
Luteinizing Hormone (LH): A hormone secreted by the anterior lobe of the pituitary. Its main function is to mature and release the egg.
Menopause: The cessation of menstruation in association with failure of the ovaries.
Metrodin: Follicle stimulating hormone.
Microsurgery: Surgery done with the assistance of the microscope, especially needed in tubal surgery because of the delicate structure and narrow opening in the tube.
Morphology of Sperm: The shape of sperm cells.
Motility: The ability of the sperm to move.
Mucous: Clear sticky fluid produced by glands around the cervix and important for transport of the sperm.
Myomectomy: An operation to remove fibroids from the uterus.
Natural Cycle: IVF or GIFT done in normal menstrual cycle.

Oestrogen: A generic term for estrus-producing compounds; the female sex hormones, including oestradiol, estriol and estrone.

Oligospermia: A reduction in sperm count from usual fertile levels (less than 20 million per ml.). In severe oligospermia there are less than 5 million per ml.

Oocyte: The egg.

Ovaries: The sexual glands of the female which produce the hormones oestrogen and progesterone and in which the eggs are developed.

Ovulation: The release of a mature egg from the ovary.

Ovum: The egg cell produced in the ovaries each month.

Pergonal: Human pituitary gonadotrophin, used to stimulate egg development and ovulation.

Peritoneal Cavity: The space inside the abdomen which contains the bowel and other vital organs, the uterus, tubes and ovaries, the liver, spleen, kidneys, gall bladder and pancreas.

Pituitary: A gland located at the base of the human brain which secretes a number of important hormones related to normal growth, development and reproduction.

Placenta: A spongy organ attached to the wall of the uterus through which nourishment and oxygen pass from the blood stream of the mother into the blood stream of the foetus through the umbilical cord.

Polyp: A fleshy swelling most often inside the uterus; it is rarely cancerous but may cause bleeding or infertility.

Post Coital Test: This determines the movement of sperm in the mucous at the neck of the womb (cervix). If the sperm do not penetrate or move in the mucous there is a barrier to conception.

Primary Infertility: The inability to conceive or carry a pregnancy to a live birth.

Progesterone: A hormone released by the ovary after ovulation. It prepares the uterine lining for embryo implantation.

Prolactin: A hormone associated with lactation. Its overproduction inhibits ovulation.

Prost: Pronuclear Stage Embryo Transfer. (early embryo)

Prostrate Gland: Situated at the base of the bladder. It with the seminal vesicles produces semen and sperm nutrients.

Rubella: A viral disease which can cause fetal abnormalities if it occurs during pregnancy - the brain, eyes and heart may be affected.

Secondary Infertility: Having before achieved a pregnancy and now unable to do so again.

Semen: The sperm and seminal secretions ejaculated during orgasm.
Semen Analysis: The study of fresh semen under the microscope to count the number, movement, the shape of the sperm. A check is made for infection and antibodies.
Sperm (spermatozoa): The male reproductive cell. Male reproductive cells are produced in the testes.
Spina Bifida: A malformation of the spine that may be associated with spinal paralysis and other abnormalities.
Split Ejaculate: A method of collecting a semen specimen so that the first half of the ejaculate is caught in one container and the rest in a second container. The first half may contain the vast majority of the sperm. The first half can then be used to inseminate the woman in appropriate cases.
Sterility: An absolute barrier to conception.
Stimulated Cycle: IVF or GIFT done in an artificial cycle, injections being used to produce several eggs.
Syngamy: The fusion of the male and female pronucleus in the egg. This occurs at about 22 hours and results in the joining of the chromosomes from the sperm and egg.
Test: Tubal Embryo Stage Transfer.
Testicle: The male sexual glands. The two are contained in the scrotum and they produce the male hormone testosterone which in turn produce the male reproductive cells, the sperm.
Testosterone: The most potent male sex hormone; produced in the testicles.
Ultrasound: Physical energy used to reflect from the body, producing images e.g. uterus, foetus, ovaries, cysts.
Umbilicus: Where the cord between the mother and foetus joins the foetus - nicknamed the 'belly button'.
Urethra: The passage that carries urine from the bladder and also carries semen from the prostate to the point of ejaculation during intercourse.
Urologist: A doctor who specialises in diseases of the urinary tract in both men and women, and also the genital organs in men.
Uterus: The organ in which the developing foetus is carried and nourished.
Vagina: The passage from the vulva to the uterus.
Vaginismus: A spasm of the muscles around the opening of the vagina, making penetration on sexual intercourse either impossible or very painful.

Varicocele: A varicose vein of the testicles which can cause male infertility.
Vas Deferens: A pair of thick-walled tubes about 45cm long in the male that lead from the epididymis to the ejaculatory duct in the prostate.
Vasectomy: Sterilizing the male by tying the vas deferens which conveys sperm from the testes to the penis.
Zift: Zygote (early embryo) Intra Fallopian Transfer.
Zona: The shell of the egg.

SUPPORT GROUPS

AUSTRALIA AND NEW ZEALAND

Infertility Federation of Australasia
PO Box 426, Erindale Centre
Wanniassa ACT 2903
Australia
Contact: Jennie (06) 291 6341

VICTORIA

IVF Friends
GPO Box 482G
Melbourne Vic 3001
Contact: Susan O'Brien (03) 437 1810

Concern
PO Box 125
Vermont Vic 3133
Contact: Anne (03) 703 1179

Endometriosis Association—Victoria
37 Andrew Crescent
South Croydon Vic 3136
Contact: Lorraine (03) 879 1276

NEW SOUTH WALES

Concern
PO Box 1347
Parramatta NSW 2150
Contact: Bob and Janine (02) 484 3769

IF Group (IVF)
C/- 13 Chiltern Road
Willoughby NSW 2068
Contact: Carol (02) 540 2226, Jenny (02) 623 1868

WESTERN AUSTRALIA

Concern for the Infertile Couple
PO Box 412
Subiaco WA 6008
Office: (08) 278 7700

QUEENSLAND

Friends of Queensland Fertility Group
PO Box 1271
Brisbane QLD 4001
Contact: Julie (07) 353 2948

JABS—S.E. QLD IVF Support Group
PO Box 6210
Upper Mt Gravatt QLD 4122

TASMANIA

ENCOMPASS
PO Box 32
North Hobart TAS 7002
Contact: Julie (002) 72 5993

AUSTRALIAN CAPITAL TERRITORY

Concern
PO Box 232
Erindale Centre
Wanniassa ACT 2903
Contact: John and Wendy (06) 291 6415

NORTHERN TERRITORY

IF Infertility Support Group
PO Box 160
Palmerston NT 0831
Contact: Elizabeth (089) 32 2421

APPROVED REPRODUCTIVE TECHNOLOGY CLINICS

QUEENSLAND

Wesley Hospital, Brisbane
(07) 371 8677, (07) 371 8246

Queensland Fertility Group, Brisbane
(07) 832 4262

Townsville Fertility Group, Townsville
Dr Glenn Schaeffer (077) 75 4490

Allamanda Infertility Medical Centre
150 Queen Street, Southport

VICTORIA

Infertility Medical Centre
Epworth Hospital, Erin Street, Richmond
(03) 429 9188

Reproductive Biology Unit
Royal Women's Hospital
132 Grattan Street, Carlton
(03) 347 6522, (03) 344 2467

Dr Jeremy Oats
Mercy Hospital, East Melbourne

Melbourne IVF
320 Victoria Parade
East Melbourne
(03) 417 3444

NEW SOUTH WALES

Royal North Shore Hospital, St Leonards
(02) 438 7027, (02) 439 8189

Royal Hospital for Women, Paddington
(02) 389 5065

St George Fertility Service
(02) 587 6343

Sydney IVF, Macquarie Street, Sydney
(02) 232 5055

King George V/Royal Alfred Hospital
Missenden Road, Camperdown

Integrated Fertility Services
12 Caroline Street, Westmead
(02) 689 1966

Infertility Clinic, Westmead

Lingard Hospital, Merewether (Newcastle)
(049) 69 3907

Albury Reproductive Medicine Clinic
1118 Pemberton Street, Albury 2640
(060) 41 2677

AUSTRALIAN CAPITAL TERRITORY

John James Memorial Hospital
Strickland Crescent, Deakin
(06) 282 5458

SOUTH AUSTRALIA

Flinders Medical Centre, Adelaide
(08) 275 9225

Queen Elizabeth Hospital, Adelaide

WESTERN AUSTRALIA

Concept (In Vitro Private)
King Edward Memorial Hospital, Subiaco
(09) 381 9559

PIVET Medical Centre (Not accredited 1989/90)
Cambridge Private Hospital, Wembley
(09) 381 9854

TASMANIA

St Helen's Hospital, Hobart
(002) 30 0850

NEW ZEALAND

Fertility Associates,
Auckland, New Zealand

North Shore Fertility,
Auckland, New Zealand

Infertility Clinic
National Women's Hospital
Auckland, New Zealand

IVF Otago
Dunedin, New Zealand

Wellington Women's Hospital
Wellington, New Zealand

Christchurch Donor Insemination Clinic
Christchurch, New Zealand

INDEX

abnormality; hormone, 16; chromosomal 61, 111
abortion rate; 11, 69, 83, 103
abstinence; 17, 27
adhesions, endometriosis 13; tubal disease, 14, 24-25
adoption; 1, 49; infertility and 88; donor egg and 99; surrogacy and 101
age; pregnancy and 8, 79, 81, 83-84; treatment and, 28; embryo and 34, 64
AIDS; test 32, 52, 95, 98-99
alcohol; effect on 17, 19, 53
amenorrhoea; 110
amniocentesis; 47, 110
anaesthetic; laparoscopy, 13, 24; egg pick-up 58; transfer 68; GIFT 71, 83
anovulation; 13, 110
antibiotics; 11, 14, 17
antibodies; 17, treatment 19-20; testing of 26, 29, 32, 52, 60, 95
anxiety; 19; about transfer 66, 69, 83; myths cause 85, 88; counselling for 92-93
artificial insemination; 18, 20, 110
aspermia; 110

basal temperature chart; 110
biopsy; 25; embryos and 61, 103
birth; 10-12; statistics and 33; risks 84; myths 86; surrogacy and 101
blastocyst; 112
bleeding; excessive 14; during embryo transfer 36, 63, 67-68

blood tests; for treatment 10; tests for infertility 18; treatment cycle and 52, 54, 64, 75; pregnancy and 81; patient requirements and 95
BOOST/FLARE; explanation of 73-74
bromocriptine; 16, 21
buserelin; 46, 54, 56, 73-79

cancer drugs; 18
capacitation; 59, 70
catheter; use of 14; embryo transfer and 67-68; during treatment 70-71
cervix; infertility 10-11, 19; tests 23-25; embryo transfer and 63, 67-68; pregnancy and 87
childlessness; 86, 89
chromosomes; 7; tests and abnormalities 29, 61, 65, 106
cilia; 111
Clomiphene; 16, 21, 73-76
cloning; 108
coitus; 23, 88
condom; 11, 17, 70
consent; legal requirement of 34, 64; counselling for 91, 95, 99
contraception; 12, 103
contracts; 68
corpus luteum; 111, 113
Cortisone; 17, 20
cost; 35-36, 65; critics of 106, 108
counselling; 8; before treatment 20; for freezing 31; questions about 32, 52-53, 91-96
cryopreservation; 6-7

culture; 2–6, 56; egg 59–60; embryo fluid 62; embryo transfer 68
curettage; 12, 24–25
custody; battle for 99–100
cysts; 13–16, 24–25, 55–56, 63, 66

Danocrine; 15
depression; 88–89
diathermy; 15, 24
donation; frozen embryos and 65; sperm and 94–95; embryos 98; law and 100
down regulation; 56, 73–74
Down's Syndrome; 8, 66
dysmenorrhoea; 112
dyspareunia; 112

ectopic pregnancy; 53, 69, 81–82
egg; IVF history 4–9; infertility 17–22; IVF, Gift and 28–30; collecting of 54; pick-up 57–58, 73–74; culture 69; fertilisation 60, 79–80; mature 62–63; freezing 65–66; Gamete 69; transfer of 80–83; donors 94
ejaculation; 17–19, 59, 70
embryo; growth and development 13, 28–29, 52–54; freezing 31, 33–34, 36, 63–65; implantation of 56; assessment and care of 61; transfer 64–70; drugs 73; pregnancy 80–83; law 102–104, critics 106–109
endometriosis; 12, 15
endometrium; 12, 15
epidural anaesthetic; 48, 68
Epworth hospital; 6, 11, 51, 120
erection; 113

Fallopian tubes; 11–12, 24, 34, 69–71
fatigue; 19
fertility; male problems with 17; effects on 19–24; reduced 30; myths about 86, 88–90
fertility drugs; 16, 73–75
fertilisation; 59–63; infertility 17, 21–22; IVF and GIFT 28–29, 70; embryos 34; treatment cycle 52–54
fibroids; 14–15, 25, 55
fimbriae; 14
flushing; 14, 57
foetus; 52–53, 81–83
follicle; failure to ovulate 13; tests for 22–25; treatment 52–55; drugs to stimulate growth 54; egg pick-up 57–58

follicle stimulating hormone (FSH); 16, 74–78
freezing; 31; embryos 36, 63–65; eggs 70

general anaesthesia; 58
general practitioner; 10
genes; 111–112
GIFT; infertility and 8, 20–22; endometriosis and 15; when to proceed to 28–31; questions about 33–34, 36–38; treatment 54, 61; procedure 69–71, 79–83
Gonadotrophin releasing hormone; 75
grief; 93

haemophilia; 103
health insurance; 35, 106–108
hormone disorders; 74; pituitary 78
hospital stay; 33–36, 38; for treatment, 64–68; myths about 86–89
hot flushes; 74
Human Chorionic Gonadotrophin (HCG); 75–77, 113
Human Menopausal Gonadotrophin (HMG) 73–76, 78
humegon; 113
hydrosalpinx; 113
hydrotubation; 14, 113
hysterosalpingogram; 23, 113

idiopathic infertility; 21–22, 113
implantation; 25, 31, 56, 66–68, 71, 98, 105
impotence; 20, 113
infection; 106; infertility and 10–14, 17–18, 26; tubal damage 29; tests for 32
infertility; causes of 10–29; questions about 32; treatment of 69, 72; pregnancy rates 79, 83; myths about 85–89; counselling for 91–95; surrogacy and 100–102
Infertility (Medical Procedures) Act; 91, 98–102, 107–108
injections; 74
injury; 99
insemination; 17–21, 110–114, 122; fertilisation and 60–61; myths about 89; counselling for 94
intercourse; 9, 25–26, 69–70, 112–113; infertility and 10–11; myths about 85–88

Index

intrauterine device (IUD); 11
in vitro fertilisation (IVF); history of 1-9; pregnancy and 28-30; egg collection for 28-30; when to proceed to 28-31; questions about 32-38; treatment cycle for 53-69; drugs and 73-78; pregnancy rates 79-84; counselling for 91-96; facts about 97-103; answering the critics of 104-109

Johnston, Mr Ian, 2
Kirkman; 101-102
Kremer test; 26, 114

lactation; 115
laparoscopy; 24, 71, 114
Leeton Prof John; 2, 10-11, 101-102
Lopata Dr Alex; 2-3, 10
lucrin; 111, 114
Lupron; 73-77
Luteal Phase Support; 77
Luteinising hormone (LH); 16, 74-75, 79, 114

malformation; 84, 116
marriage; 97, 99
masturbation; 27, 70, 72
media; 9, 50, 60, 79, 89, 104
menopause; 7-8, 13, 30, 43, 73, 114
menstrual cycle; 4, 8, 16, 23, 63, 111, 112, 114
menstruation; 16, 110-114
metrodin; 56, 73-75, 78
microsurgery; 1, 14, 20
miscarriage; 30, 45, 53, 69, 81, 114
mucous; 23, 88; hormones and 16-17, 21; testing 25-26; egg pick-up and 57, 60; egg transfer and 68
multiple pregnancy; 16, 33-34, 47, 62, 82-83, 105
muscular dystrophy; 112

natural cycle; 5, 8, 31, 56, 64

oestrogen; 8-9, 15, 22, 25, 64, 75, 81
oligospermia; 115
ovaries; 3-16, 21; surgery and 30-31; during treatment cycle 54-58; egg transfer and 62-66; drugs and 74
ovulation; 4-16, 21-23, 54-55, 57-59, 64, 87-88, 104, 110; stimulation of 74
ovum; 70, 107, 115

pain; 11-14, 16, 69-70, 72
penis; 87, 112, 117
Pelvic Inflammatory Disease (PID); 11-12
Pill; 5, 11, 85
pituitary gland; 75-78, 112-113
placenta; 9, 113-115
pregnancy; 2-6, 101-105; and fertility 19-23; IVF, GIFT and 28-31; questions about 28-31; treatment cycle and 52-54, 62-65; blood tests for 56, 69; rates of 71, 79-83; myths about 86-87; counselling 94-97
progesterone; 8-9, 15-16, 22, 25, 56, 64, 75-78,
progestogens; 15
prolactin; 13, 16, 21-22, 52
PROST; 29, 115
psychological; 51, 88

Queen Victoria Medical Centre; 2-7, 10, 13, 50

rejection; 2
relaxation; 48, 93
Royal Women's Hospital; 2-4, 10-13, 120
rubella; 32, 52, 95, 115

Sathananthan; 5
scrotum; 19, 113, 116
selection; 60
semen analysis; 10, 21, 26-27, 32, 52, 86-87, 116
semen sample; 17
sexual intercourse; 11, 69, 85-86, 116
smoking, 17-19, 53
speculum; 67
sperm antibodies; 20, 26, 29, 32, 52, 95
sperm count; 88, 97, 115
sperm donation; 95
sperm movement; 10, 111
sperm production; 18-19, 112
sperm quality; 19, 27, 34, 62
spina bifida; 30, 84, 116
Steptoe; 2-4, 10
sterility; 10, 116
stress; 13, 17-19, 50, 69, 80, 88-89, 92-93, 105
sub-fertility; 10
support groups; 49, 51, 118
surgery; 14-15, 19, 24, 29, 39, 82-84, 94, 106, 110-114

surrogacy; 101, 107

temperature chart; 23, 86, 110
Tubal embryo stage transfer (TEST); 29, 36
testes; 18-19, 112, 116-117
testosterone; 18, 22, 116
triplets, 32, 62, 82-83, 99
Trounson Dr Alan; 2-4, 6-7, 10-11
tubal disease; 10-11, 14, 21, 28, 79, 82
tubal surgery; 1, 29, 83, 114
twins; 11, 62, 82-83, 108

ultrasound; 13, 25, 35, 38, 54-58, 67-69, 71, 81, 84, 95, 116
undescended testes; 18

uterus; infertility and 12-15, 19; tests 23-25; lining of 31; embryo transfer 54, 66-69; egg collection 58; fertilisation 61-63; pregnancy and 81-83

vagina; 17-19, 23, 57, 67-68, 71, 87, 111, 116
vasectomy; 11, 18, 117

waiting list; 6, 31, 33, 53, 72, 81
World Health Organisation; 106

X-ray; 23, 113

Zygote intra fallopian tube (ZIFT) 29, 117